CW00422133

Strictly for Therapists

causes, effects and strategies
for effective treatment
with hypnotherapy,
and NLP

by

John Smale DHP BA(Hons)

STRICTLY FOR THERAPISTS

Published in July 2009 by emp3books Ltd
Kiln Workshops, Pilcot Road, Crookham Village,
Fleet, Hampshire, GU51 5RY, England

©John Smale 2009

The author asserts then moral right to be identified as the author of this work. All views are those of the author.

ISBN-10: 0-9550736-9-3
ISBN-13: 978-0-9550736-9-4

All rights reserved. No part of this publication may be reproduced, stored in a retrieval system, or transmitted, in any form or by any means, electronic, mechanical, photocopying, recording or otherwise without the prior written consent of the author.

Limit of Liability/ Disclaimer of Warranty. Whilst the author and publisher have used their best efforts in preparing this book, they make no representation or warranties with respect to the accuracy or completeness of this book and specifically disclaim any warranties of completeness or saleability or fitness of purpose. The advice given in this book may not be suitable for your specific situation and is offered for guidance. The publisher is not offering professional services and you should consult a professional where appropriate. Neither the author nor the publisher shall be liable for any damages, including but not limited to special, incidental, consequential or any other damages.

www.emp3books.com

Other publications by the author include:

Short Stories and Metaphors
ISBN: 978-0-9550736-3-2

The Secret Language of Hypnotherapy
ISBN: 978-0-9550736-2-5

Mind Changing Short Stories and Metaphors
ISBN: 978-0-9550736-4-9

More information from:
http://www.emp3books.com

STRICTLY FOR THERAPISTS

**dedicated to all therapists who work
to give their clients an improved
quality of life**

STRICTLY FOR THERAPISTS

CONTENTS

Introduction

Strictly for Therapists is an honest and open book that explains the causes, effects and treatments for many of the problems that a therapist is asked to deal with. Very often therapy is similar to doing a cryptic crossword. You have to look for clues from your clients but this book helps you by giving a lot of the letters for you to make solving those puzzles easier. The task is to expose the cause, defuse the negative effects of that cause and then to build a positive future for your clients. They will trust you to help; this book helps you to help.

A therapist is a catalyst for beneficial change. He/she listens, and then works out patterns and then changes perceptions to achieve constructive results. He/she should be a facilitator for positive change rather than a creator of a Frankenstein client full of false beliefs. A therapist is a channel for change. End of story.

The following book is an appraisal of the author's experiences with a large number of problems presented by many clients over a substantial period of time. It is aimed at giving guidance and sensible advice to new therapists, established therapists and their clients.

When I started as a therapist, my first few years of practice were based on the training I had received. This gave a foundation to my work but the therapy became elongated rather than efficient. The expectations of outcomes that had been prescribed were different in practice.

The conflicts that we hold in our minds are often those between the primeval, instinctual parts and the stresses and demands of modern life. The real clash, then, is that between the basic natures of mankind in contrast to the rules we feel we have to follow as a species that is crowded onto a planet that has changed from those old times.

When I am asked which problems I help to resolve, the answer is easy; two. Yes, two! This is because I deal with the two primeval survival systems that emerge in different forms, namely the 'fight or flight' response and our ability to store fat.

However, the ways in which they show themselves are varied. This book tells you how to recognise their different guises and how to resolve the underlying problems.

Small parts in this book have been abbreviated and adapted from The Secret Language of Hypnotherapy. It seems foolish to withhold methods from therapists who can use them to great effect with their clients. These include some weight control methods plus breathing, posture and language techniques. Where those extracts have been included they have been modified to suit usage by therapists.

What you will be doing, as a therapist, is reconciling the basic primeval drives that we continue to hold with a totally different set of circumstances in modern life. Those reactions keep an insomniac awake as they live on a hair-trigger that would have warned of a lion prowling around outside. It makes us want to escape from dangers, real or perceived as in panic attacks. It makes us become threatening and angry when confronted by situations that could be dealt with by more 'civilised' methods. It can make us store excess fat when under stressful conditions. And so on.

This book cuts away some of the absurdities in complicated therapy and allows the therapist to offer sound and constructive help in achieving a positive outcome for the client.

So what follows is in the best interest of therapists and clients alike. Efficiency never reduces outcomes; instead it increases the reputation of the therapist. The book gives broad hints as to cause and effect but it never supposes that they will always fit the circumstances or problem of the client. You, the therapist, have to do the hard work and never assume you know the answers.

Ethics are essential. Honesty and the achievement of best practice are vital.

PART ONE

The Client

The most important things in your practice are your clients. Treat them with honesty, high ethics and good care.

The Introductory Consultation

When your clients arrive for their first appointments, shake hands and direct them to their seat. Shaking hands is the only way in which you should ever touch them. Hugging during tears is absolutely forbidden. As the therapist you are offering to be trusted and any gesture other than shaking hands, politely, is to be absolutely avoided.

The introductory consultation does a few things. First, and above all, it should evaluate the problem so that you, as the therapist, feel competent to handle it. Clients are there for help rather than as experiments or for the therapist's training. So there is a chicken and egg situation here. How does a therapist gain experience so that he or she can handle a variety of conditions?

The only answer is to work with and discuss, at length, the scenarios that are likely to be presented when you are training. Thereafter, this involves the use of 'supervision' whereby a therapist can talk about individual cases to somebody who has broader experience and knowledge. This is so necessary. When we consider that a poor attempt at treatment by an inexperienced therapist can cause an incredible amount of damage, it is vital that the therapist is knowledgeable and competent to help.

Taking that as read, then the introductory consultation should gain as much information as possible before committing the client to a course of treatment.

Never make assumptions or jump to conclusions. I remember meeting a member of an association when I was training. He looked at my green watchstrap and made his decision about what my issues with life were without a question. He told me that he knew the cause of every problem, including mine, within 30 seconds of meeting a client!

What he never asked was why I was wearing a green leather watchstrap; he assumed he knew why; some deep psychological hang-up, I am sure he thought. Well, the answer is that I worked as the Marketing Director of one of the largest producers of high quality watchstraps at the time. I was wearing it because it advertised my company's style and quality to our customers. I never told him because he never asked.

At the start, ask the client permission to take written notes and get a signature to avoid breaching the Data Protection Act 1998. It is worth reading the Act or the equivalent laws in different countries. They are available by searching the Internet. Always keep files in a totally secure place and shred them when treatment is finished to the satisfaction of the client.

With a pen and paper you are able to write notes and watch the client for clues at the same time. Experience tells you how to read body language and to see visual clues. There are some good books about body language that you should read.

I have never seen the point of storing information on computer files. Recording of information is best done using a pen and paper. Tape recordings, digital audio files and videos need to be listened to or watched. How do you find the time, and how would you give better service by recording? It also runs a legal gauntlet in the protection of data.

I also feel that wiring up a client or setting up a video camera (weird!) gives the impression of wanting control. I think the desire to video record sessions is very close to being voyeuristic. Everybody that a therapist sees is controlled by their problem. To give the impression of control, as a stage hypnotist does, will work against treatment rather than help to resolve the issue.

Dress codes should include looking like a sympathetic character rather than like a control figure such as a bank manager or head-teacher. This extends to the layout of an office. A woman who has been sexually abused will react against a couch that looks as if it should belong in a gynaecologist's office.

When meeting the client, the process is similar to 'cold reading', practised by street magicians and pseudo-psychics but a therapist does it for pure information rather than to impress. Look for visible bruises, hangovers, wedding or engagement rings and whether or not the client makes eye contact. Also scan, discreetly, for scars from acne or eczema. These might have been the cause of verbal bullying when they were younger. See if the body is in a relaxed or anxious position, check if the breathing is high or low, whether sentences used in speech are long with a sharp intake of breath or relaxed and a whole lot more. This will become equally relevant when taking information.

I always start with the question, "How can I help you?" You are there to help and this statement should be made at the beginning. The client should then tell you. You should be writing notes from the outset before taking personal information. Watch for emotion from the whole spectrum. Laughter that seems inappropriate should be noted. Tears should be responded to by the handing over of a tissue whilst remembering and noting what preceded them.

The client might give a precise summary or a seemingly never-ending description. It is too easy to interrupt but the job of a therapist is to listen. If the client is talking then it might be because they have never had anybody they can talk to without interruption, advice or judgement.

When they have come to a suitable point, ask them for their personal details. You need their name, address, telephone number, date of birth and age as a matter of routine. If they wish to keep knowledge of their treatment away from family members ensure you have a mobile telephone number so that if the client needs to be contacted you can make a discreet call. You will only call a client if you have an emergency and need to change an appointment.

Their occupation is important as it shows the therapist a life style. A single mother who works a long day has a different view of life to an heiress who lives in a stately home. Somebody who is a high–flyer is stressed in a different way as they are perpetually making choices between family and work.

Then ask for the client's marital status. This will tell you about how they live. It will tell you about divorces and partnerships. When they are in a relationship, ask how long it has been for. If they have split, ask them when it was and what the reasons were. Find out about the relationship with an 'ex' after a split.

Sexuality should never be asked. If the client is gay or lesbian, they will volunteer the information.

Ask about children and how old they are. You will gain details of step-children or a partner's children. In this case ask with whom the children live.

Then ask if the client has, or has had, brothers and/or sisters. The 'has had' will bring to light any siblings who have died. Find out how that happened. Sibling relationships also shows the dynamics of half and step-siblings. It shows the family position of the client in their childhood situation. (See the chapter on Siblings for more information.)

Key information is given when you ask 'Who brought you up?' This tells about past and present relationships with parents, their divorces and infidelities, whether or not they are alive, and so on.

Therapy involves a huge web of dynamics. It is necessary to know what is involved at the outset. If the problem is beyond your skills, you must refer them to somebody else with more experience. The professional societies and associations will provide this information. And if, during information gathering you feel that you are being 'nosy' or impolite, then you will have chosen the wrong profession to work in!

Ask when the problem began, but inwardly, be open minded. Often somebody will tell you a few months ago and then, on further questioning, they will tell you it was many years ago. Nobody will tell a doctor that they have ignored a lump or bump for ages at first telling through feeling embarrassed about failing to seek advice or treatment earlier. It is the same for deep emotional problems.

Also, find out how the client heard about you. This will hone your advertising/marketing efforts. If they heard about you from a friend or colleague, **never** talk about the third party. This, number one, confirms that their acquaintance saw you for therapy and, number two, it will totally obliterate your promise of confidentiality.

You should discuss your terms at an appropriate moment. They probably asked you for information when they made the appointment, but you and the client should be clear on the payment detail.

I ask for payment one session in advance. Rather than for greed, because you actually make no more money by doing this, it ensures that the client will arrive for the first session. And it requests commitment from the client. After the client has paid and you have their appointment in your diary, you can teach them some relaxation techniques. They need to walk away feeling that the first step to their recovery has been taken. In fact, it has. Many clients will report feeling better after their first meeting because they have spoken to somebody who is neutral and who has listened without giving reaction or advice.

The following is a small scale copy of the form I use for client information. To use it, the therapist should use the headings and columns on their own form using A4 paper, leaving enough space to make full notes.

STRICTLY CONFIDENTIAL CLIENT INFORMATION

Advertising source	Date	Fee
NAME		
ADDRESS		
TELEPHONE Mobile		
Date of birth AGE		
OCCUPATION		
MARITAL STATUS		
CHILDREN		
AGES AND SEXES OF SIBLINGS		
RAISED BY		
PROBLEM		
When started:		
(continued overleaf)		

4X4 (more of this later)
X RELAX (more of this later)

I give permission to ………………………………. (your name) to make confidential personal written notes during the course of my therapy.

Signed……………………………………..

Print name………………………………..

Dated………………………………………..

Sometimes clients recognise the phrase 'adrenaline rush', but it is surprising how many people that I have seen have never heard the term 'fight or flight' response that is the cause of so many problems. However, those two terms, fight and flight are active responses. That is, when under threat, the person wants to fight the cause or run away from it.

Yet there are two passive responses, those of defending and freezing.

Anxious clients are defending and freezing at the same time so it is a good idea to open dialogue as quickly as possible to get them to relax. 'Opening up' is about them describing their problem whilst opening up their tight body posture.

One of the things I look for in clients who need help for stress, anxiety and panic is their speech pattern.

WATCHING THE BREATHING

The diagram that follows shows anxious breathing. People who are anxious will often speak long sentences, rapidly and with short sharp intakes of breath. This means that they are using just the upper part of their chests to breathe and this leads to a form of hyperventilation, which leads to anxiety and panic. (See the chapter titled **Breathing**.)

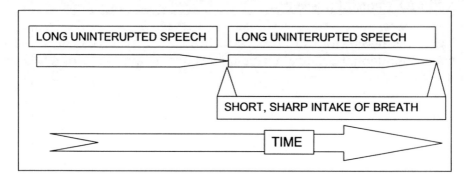

If you hold your breath for as long as it takes your client to breathe between their long dialogues, you will start to feel uncomfortable!

You are a therapist so your profession is offering effective help to your clients. One simple thing to do is to point out the bad breathing pattern. Get them to breathe in a deep and slow way using their diaphragms. They need to stop between sentences for a breath as if commas and full stops were cues to breathe.

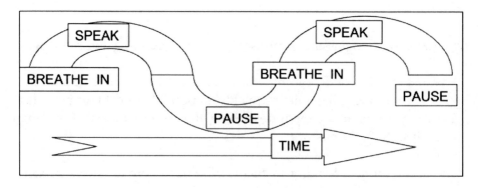

There should be a pause in speech, a deep inward breath and then a resumption of speech in a slow and calm way as the diagram above shows.

Another thing that I look for is their body position. They will often have their arms crossed at the wrists and legs crossed at the ankles. This is closed body language, but most of all it is a defensive pose.

Note Taking

There is no point in taking notes if you fail to read them before a new session!

I record what the client says as close to verbatim as possible. It is important to be able to see language clues at later points. This wording gives the therapist direction. For example, if a client talks about something, they might use a colouring word. Such a word might be "My world crashed around me" spoken by a flying phobic talking about a relationship that ended on a holiday. This is referred to as 'sub literal language', the language that is unconsciously chosen to express something. It is similar to visual body language in that respect. I then underline the words.

I use symbols in circles for ease of quick reference for various things:

U means 'upset'.
T means 'tears'.
VUT means very upset and with tears.
B means 'blushing'.
And so on. You can devise your own for other things.

If I ask a question then I put it in square brackets, for example [EARLIEST?] This question often opens a client's recall if they are hesitant to start or if they get stuck and go blank.

At the end of a session I make notes about what has happened, hypotheses that I have and actions, if any, for the next session. You should refrain from discussing session content with the client as this can lead him/her in a direction that is incorrect.

Your notes are a log of the treatment and progress of the client. Write them as you go and read them after the session and again before the next session. I have a thirty minute break between clients to read notes, return phone calls, write replies to emails and to relax.

Testimonials

I am a fantastic therapist who achieves perfect results with every client. To prove the point I will advertise or add to my web pages testimonials from happy clients, real or fictional.

WRONG

In the first place you will never help everybody that you see. That dream is never achievable. Secondly, unnamed testimonials can be, and often are, made up. Testimonials that have names attached have been solicited from clients. The issues here are that named testimonials tell prospective clients that your promise of confidentiality is hokum and that you lack enough self-belief that you have to use strange tactics to get business.

Perfect results are impossible so if you boast about successes then you should also declare failures.

Claims for stop-smoking successes always amuse me. 95% success rate! How is success measured? Is it for one day, one week, one month, one year or a lifetime? Do therapists continually telephone clients to ask if they are still non-smokers? Any figure you see claiming high success rates needs to be questioned in detail. Any therapist who uses them runs a huge risk of misleading clients.

The other classic is the use of celebrity names. I have seen many high-flying people in entertainment, the media, Government and business over the years. The idea of letting slip a single name or position is absolutely beyond my principles and ethics.

However, I have a huge number of postcards from flying phobics pinned to boards in my office. They only show locations and never names. This is done to offer hope to new flying phobics rather than to boast and make unreasonable claims.

Promises and Guarantees

Never, but never, promise to help somebody because you hope you might be able to. Only take on a client when you are sure that you can help. The outcome, otherwise, is that you have given false hope for the fees you will earn rather than for offering genuine treatment.

It is also pointless to promise that the client's problem will be resolved in a set number of sessions. You can give an indication of the number it will take, but the client and you will find areas that need to be explored and resolved. Even if you work to prescribed therapy systems that tell you what to do session by session, ask yourself how a generalised system can always be the right one for each problem you will encounter.

Guarantees are equally foolish. There will be clients who you are unable to help. This may be you or it may be them. You will never, ever, be able to promise that a client's problem will be resolved. If you give a guarantee that they will get better then you are misleading people who need to be told in honest terms what you can offer.

In the same area, when you promise a smoker a second or third session at half-price, or for free, then you should be aware that you are suggesting that they might need more sessions than those you offer or you build a safety net that is actually dangerous.

'I can have a cigarette or two because if I get hooked again I can go back to see the therapist for free so it is worth the risk.'

I never answer the question, 'what if I do not give up?' I will truthfully tell the enquirer that I never hear the word 'if'. You may think that is offering a promise that is unable to be met, or that I offer a guarantee. Look at the words again. If pushed, I will tell people that stopping smoking is a percentage game. I will explain that some people will continue smoking after therapy, but most will stop. This is nothing more than the truth.

Should a client need more than one session I charge my normal fee. There is no reason why I should give a discount. This could just be the reason that a hesitant quitter starts again. I must incentivise my clients to stop by offering a penalty rather than an inducement.

With all therapy, the best way to get results is to work within the bounds of your knowledge. Keep learning and honing your skills and techniques. Avoid being tempted into weird and wonderful therapies that offer to make you richer and able to charge more for their style of treatment. If they are making promises that they are unable to substantiate, or that other therapists have seen through, they are fooling you by selling fool's gold.

STRICTLY FOR THERAPISTS

PART TWO

Forms of Therapy

Psychotherapy, Hypnotherapy, Active Imagination, Shamanism and NLP

There are common roots which connect therapies. These methods need not be mutually exclusive and a 'cocktail' of different approaches is sometimes necessary. We should avoid working within fixed frames. We should have an eclectic approach to the way in which we, as therapists, should work.

Those systems include psychotherapy, hypnotherapy, active imagination, shamanism and NLP

The core theme of those different approaches to therapy is the method of communication with the unconscious mind. Coming to terms with the unconscious mind seems to be at the root of all of the processes involved.

It becomes necessary to present an assumption that the unconscious mind is represented as different models within the context of each approach, but that the underlying processes of unconscious thought are universal. There is also the assumption that the unconscious mind is separate to the conscious mind and that they are not necessarily on the same wavelength!

As part of an overview I will now summarise the aims of the different approaches ahead of a broader explanation of the individual methods.

Psychotherapy is a collective term for creating mental well-being with clients with mental (emotional) problems. It encompasses a wide range of techniques from analysis, behavioural change and facilitating interpersonal communication. The following are some of the methods therapists will use.

For hypnotherapy the underlying aim is to elicit the responses of the unconscious to bring about changes in the entire organism that cannot be brought about by conscious will. This is done by either making changes to the current thinking process, or by reconciling past trauma in order to allow a fundamental change in those thinking processes.

Jung's methodology was to bring about those changes by listening to the activities of the unconscious mind and thereby bringing about reconciliation of conflict. Hypnosis aims to do the same thing by both listening to, and directly communicating changes to, the unconscious.

NLP is a different way to view and influence the unconscious by observing and using the different communication modalities which are influenced and directed by the unconscious.

The aims of shamanism are to enjoy the experiences of a wider world, a spiritual one which, I propose, is in fact a construct of the unconscious mind, in order to learn and change. This element of the 'deeper' world is present in Jung's collective unconscious.

There are differences in the approaches which involve passivity. Shamanism is very passive with somebody else, usually, taking responsibility for the communication with the 'other world' for 'healing', therapy.

Active imagination allows the unconscious to take over the thought processes, but is an individual activity, even if directed by a therapist.

Hypnosis relies on the therapist. (I believe that the effects of self-hypnosis are different to those of directed hypnosis, simply because in self-hypnosis the conscious mind is offering subjective direction which allows the resistances which hide trauma to operate. This view may be substantiated by the lack of examples, if any, where successful self-help by using such methods for fundamental changes is claimed).

NLP is usually about working problems out with another person when used in a therapeutic context. When NLP is used as a self-help technique, it is similar to self-hypnosis in that positive thoughts and suggestions can be made and acted upon, but it needs an objective helper when used for therapies which need fundamental changes.

In short, NLP considers man's communication with man in the present time in order to allow positive change for the future. Hypnotherapy considers man's communication with man to recall events from the past in order to allow change for the future (analysis), and communication in the present for positive change in the future (suggestion).

Jung's active imagination considers man's communication with man and the inherent images which are assumed to be present in every man, and their reconciliation, with the intention of change.

Shamanism considers man's resolution with the influences of a different, usually invisible, world of spirits (the unconscious), in order to bring about healing.

I will explain the four modalities in the order of Shamanism; Jung's active imagination as a 'modern' marriage of psychotherapy with older beliefs; hypnosis as a psychotherapeutic technique and, finally, NLP as a use of hypnosis and many other techniques.

SHAMANISM.
This seems at first glance to be a strange subject to include in this book. However, rather than being promoted as a therapy in its own right, it is included as one of the building blocks of what we do. Shamanism is relevant to the way in which analytical therapists work. Most of our problems come from our submerged primeval past. It seems right to consider how those problems were, and are, treated.

Shamanism is a tradition spanning at least 50,000 years. It is an almost universal philosophy, experience, and a guiding way of life in what can only be described as older societies such as the Native American Indians, Australian aborigines, South American natives, Siberian and Eskimo communities, some African tribes and other cultures around the world.

It cannot be described as a religion as there is no concept of a God figure at the top of a power and virtue hierarchy, but rather that life itself has a shared energy which effects every different component, at almost the atomic level, so that rocks, other non-organic forms, plants and other animals are included in the 'great scheme of things'.

In shamanism, life exists on at least two levels, the 'real world' that is the hard physical world which modern society recognises, and the 'other world', which is thought to be inhabited by spirits. This other world is non-linear, non-temporal and in contemporary terms 'non-logical'. In this way it is similar to the descriptions and distinctions often made for the 'right brain' and the 'left brain' described later in the section on NLP!

This concept of this separation of the mind into two separate parts is, of course, analogous to the conscious and unconscious minds, in which the conscious is awareness and the unconscious is the hidden driver and the prime source of influence. The 'other world' is made of a lower-world, the place which is entered by, for one example, a tunnel from a cave which then opens into bright landscapes. In this world soul-retrieval can take place, finding parts of a person that have been mislaid. In this sense the lost part may be considered to be suppressed memories. The other part of the shamanic world, reached, for another example, by climbing a mountain, tree or other symbol of travelling upwards, is the upper-world, in which help and guidance may be found.

Illness is seen as separation from spirits, from nature, from the Source (the Creator and the Creation) and from the community. The role of the shaman in healing is in removing hurtful influences such as spiritual darts and/or spirits by using the beneficial influence of his, and the sufferer's, spirits during what might be described as trance-work.

People are assumed to have benevolent allies that live in the spirit world, which can be brought back into the 'real' world in order to assist in healing or personal development. These are described as power animals. (An interesting parallel theme in human history is the human/animal hybrid seen in cave paintings, old ritual dances, Greek legends such as the Minotaur and repeated in werewolf mythology). These power animals are used to both ward off, and to defeat, the harmful influences which are causing illnesses.

If we take this harmful population of the 'other world' as metaphors or symbols for trauma and other causes of conflict, and the power animals and plants as metaphors for the curative process, then the defeat of the harmful influences becomes catharsis, and resolution. This parallels the use of metaphors in hypnosis and NLP where they are, in effect, communication in the language of the unconscious mind which is based on broader foundations than verbal language alone which is the predominant mode of conscious thought.

One of the methods to access the spirit world, the unconscious mind, is by undertaking a shamanic journey. Although the shamanic journey may be taken by the individual for personal experience, the type of journey described is the healing journey taken by a shaman on behalf of another. The main constituents of a healing shamanic journey seem to be ritual, induction by drumming and speech, starting in the entrance to a cave or deep hole, a deepening process that involves moving down through a tunnel, and emergence into a different place which is bright and spacious. Then there is the introduction of a power animal or an attempt at 'soul retrieval', and a return to the 'real' world for mending. It would be naïve to assume that only the shaman is affected. The recipient of treatment will also be influenced by the whole process and ceremony. The experiences include sharp visual images, and sensations of falling or of rushing downwards. The mind is very receptive to the intensity of the episode.

At this stage it is useful to introduce some thinking on the mechanics of what is happening during this process by describing the first stages of sleep.

When we fall asleep, or enter hypnosis, beta waves in the brain decrease and the heart rate slows. Theta waves increase as we move closer to sleep when delta waves also increase.

The regular beating of a drum at a frequency of 4 to 7 beats per minute will result in an increase of theta waves.

Theta waves are also present during dreaming sleep, REM (rapid eye movement). An interesting aspect during this stage of half-wake, half-sleep, is that of *virtual paralysis*, presumably to prevent the dreamer from 'acting out' his dreams. Although there is a lot of case law that would deny that, such as when men dream that they are killing an enemy whilst strangling their wives, for example! This behaviour can occur in certain sleep disorders, however. This feeling of paralysis is something referred to by people when using hallucinogenic drugs.

If the 'state' induced by shamanic journeys is the result of a change in brain wave patterns, as happens in hypnosis and the early stages of sleep, this would give an explanation to the universal nature of the experiences. However, it then has to be assumed that there is a pool of information that the human unconscious contains at a primeval level. Instincts are based on actions, bees making honey, birds building nests, humans suckling, etc. Possibly there are also basic concepts and reactions such as mimicry, language and so on, which are not fundamental but the predisposition to learn them appears to be.

It could also be postulated that every human, and other animal, has a surreal mental construct of the world, or environment, or even animal specific culture in which it exists. This could be the area that Jung envisaged within the collective unconscious, the archetypes being culture specific but representational of key figures such as the mother.

JUNG

Jung's prime concern was resolving the conflict between the conscious and unconscious minds. In his terms, the conscious being the part with which we have an awareness of ourselves, the unconscious being the part that has different drives, including the collective unconscious, made up of instincts and archetypes. His prime concern was the reconciliation of those two parts by enabling channels of communication to be set up so that the conflicts could be brought to consciousness and thereby dealt with. Active imagination is the broad description of his methodology, but it is also taken in a narrower sense as the daydream, fantasy and dream work which he undertook.

Jung talked about the conscious mind assimilating the unconscious in order to achieve a balance at the mid-point and used as examples Christ being within the person, or of the Tao concept of the Middle Way, and to nirvana, the Buddhist concept of "the extinction of individuality and the absorption into the supreme spirit" (Concise Oxford Dictionary).

Jung made the case that the unconscious mind is the 'real' mind which is inhibited by the conscious, logical functioning. His techniques were aimed at quietening consciousness to allow a full flight of unconscious fancy. The involvement in the fantasy world which, he assumed inhabits all of us is also the aim of shamanism in whichever way it is evoked, by drugs, meditation, journeys, etc.

At some points he tried to differentiate between fantasy and imagination. However in most of his texts he used the words interchangeably. He defined active imagination as building inner images from a starting point such as staring at a picture.

Some of Jung's experiences have a great deal in common with shamanic concepts. For example he had a spirit guru, Shankaracharya, an example of an upper-world helper. He also referred to falling into a deep hole when confronting his own depression. He saw the entrance to a dark cave which led, not to landscapes, but to symbols of birth and death.

Jung was a scholar of mythology and a great number of the characters from mythology were a part of his dreaming and meditations, which tends to reinforce the assumption that the unconscious mind learns to reflect the culture of the person rather than to contain absolute figures.

The unanswered question is do we all share a common set of

unconscious images which exist in our basic genetic programming and which are modified by our experiences, and of which we are vaguely aware of through our dreams, poetry, art, fantasies and which we would like to experience with our conscious minds?

Jung's active imagination is a therapeutic technique which allows unconscious content to be exposed in a waking state. It is like "dreaming with open eyes", but unlike the passivity of dreams, it demands the active participation of the individual. The images which arise may be elaborated through artistic and self-expressive mediums such as painting.

It also included dream discussion, rather than interpretation, symbol interpretation as in old archetypal symbols, painting inner thoughts, which often resulted in a form of early symbolism.

HYPNOTHERAPY
There are three types of clients who seek out a hypnotherapist. The first are those who have seen a hypnotherapist in the past or those who have been recommended to see you by an ex-client of yours. These people have realistic expectations about the therapy.

The second are those people who have an open mind and they have perhaps heard or read that hypnotherapy can help to resolve their problems.

The third types are looking for a fast fix because they have seen a hypnotist working on the TV or stage. They need to be told that there are no such things as magical cures for their problems. This can lead to a loss of faith in your abilities, but you need to be honest in your description of your course of treatments.

I sometimes give an explanation of stage hypnotists in relation to 'magicians' in my childhood who would perform a trick and then imply that they had the knowledge of occult forces. Nowadays, magicians are illusionists who use skill and dexterity to perform their art. Nobody believes that they have a secret knowledge. Stage hypnotists sometimes adopt the first scenario of 'magic' to perform. We know that their skills are a cleverly manufactured illusion made from words and the creation of compliance.

I explain that my job is to act as a facilitator for the release of the emotional pressure that is causing a problem. I feel that I am a catalyst for change rather than an integral part of the reaction. I explain that we are wonderful in our logical world in looking for a-to-z explanations. I tell my clients that it is necessary to invent a word. Rather than rationalising a problem we have to 'emotionalise' it.

As a simplistic definition, hypnotherapy is therapy in which the phenomena of hypnosis are used!! To justify such a trite explanation, it seems to be that the phenomena of hypnosis vary with different people, and the use of hypnosis changes with differing goals.

The common thread within the different approaches, however, is the desire to obtain communication between the conscious and unconscious minds, in some cases one-way, and in others, two-way, albeit the shamanic approach is oblivious to psychological concepts of conscious and unconscious, but defines them as 'ordinary reality' and 'non-ordinary reality'.

Sometimes this communication is verbal, sometimes metaphorical (from the Greek, 'to transfer change'), a better word than symbolic, the distinction that Jung made with Freud's dream language. In one-way communication, the therapist is aiming to change the unconscious thoughts, drives and motivations so that the client will benefit from those changes without the conflict between his conscious and unconscious minds. For example the elimination of habits which are thought to be bad, but which are acted upon, nonetheless. In two-way communication, the emotional memories, values and experiences held in the unconscious mind are exhumed and dealt with by the more rational conscious mind which can interpret the emotional mis-information in a 'rational' way and re-store it in the unconscious mind without the negative or damaging associations being re-enacted when current, or future, stimuli or prompts are given.

In terms of similarity with shamanism and 'active imagination', I have worked with cases where clients have gone off into a type of active imagination, recalling fantasies which were obviously not real such as inventing scenarios which represented certain themes within their lives. I have also seen clients who were floating over a childhood home, or such like. It is interesting that a great number of these accounts involve flying or floating in the air. There are also the frequent physical feelings of floating, spinning, falling, sinking etc. mentioned as being typical of the theta state, above. Some of the hypnosis suggestibility tests include phenomena such as arm catalepsy etc., perhaps a sign of the 'virtual paralysis' mentioned above.

It is highly likely that shamanism, 'active imagination' and hypnosis are all facets of the same natural phenomena, albeit the variation in practical terms, being changes in the processes of application. I must add that I have taken a few people, with their permission and compliance, who are used to hypnosis, on what must be described as shamanic journeys. The 'induction' involved nothing more than asking them to imagine standing at the entrance to a tunnel which led down into the ground, and then asking them to describe what happened. The similarities with the descriptions of shamanic journeys that I have read were quite uncanny! They included ribbed tunnels with spiked obstacles, landscapes at the end, waterfalls, trees, ferns, animals and sound. There was a feeling of falling, usually at the far end of the tunnel, and an intense arousal of emotion when I introduced the concept of a benevolent power animal. I used relaxing hypnotherapy music rather than drums. Although this is nowhere near an objective or scientifically controlled experiment, it gives me a notion that the phenomena involved were the same as those used in hypnosis. Similarities to the phenomena of active imagination are mentioned above.

NLP
Neuro-Linguistic Programming is an application of techniques to bring about changes to a person. 'Neuro' relates to the mind and how it works, 'Linguistic' refers to the ways in which people communicate, 'Programming' refers to the analogy of the mind to the computer and

the ways in which people are assumed to have personal programmes that can be changed.

A great deal of NLP deals with effective communication, indeed an NLP definition of hypnosis is 'effective communication', using signals and clues, and to an extent, language constructions, which are unconscious in nature. For example, in the areas of body language, eye movements reflect past, present and future thoughts and feelings. It is felt that people favour different thought modalities related to their sensory systems, such as visual, auditory, and kinaesthetic. These unconscious modalities can be recognised by their use of language; 'I see what you mean', 'I hear what you're saying', 'I feel it makes sense', for example. Communication can be improved if the therapist can recognise and utilise those modalities.

The above is concerned with unconscious communication, and improved effectiveness. NLP also uses the metaphor as a more effective method of communication. The role model used for hypnotherapy is Milton H. Erickson, (1902-1980), a master of communication by direct and indirect means, such as the metaphor, analogy and example. In his model there rests the essence of beneficial change which is used by hypnotherapists. Those effective methods have been extended into other areas of life as well as those people with psychological problems. It has developed the therapeutic process into a method for changing situations which cause problems within relationships, work and within the person himself. 'Positive thinking' is necessary for therapy and also for extending and achieving personal goals. Such thinking needs an effective way for the individual to communicate with his own unconscious mind.

NLP follows the belief that the brain hemispheres are separate and have different functions, although it is also accepted that all people do not follow the same patterns and structures. The left hemisphere is considered to be the dominant one in the majority of people and contains conscious functions such as logic and language. The right hemisphere is considered to be more holistic, intuitive and concerned with visualisation, imagination and creativity. These are the qualities that are felt to belong to the unconscious mind. The argument is not substantiated other than in the location of language and speech functions but, notwithstanding the argument about where the conscious and unconscious minds reside, the distinction between conscious and unconscious definitions, functions and qualities seems to be valid.

There are key areas within NLP that seem to be based on Erickson's methodology and have to some extent been renamed in NLP jargon. These are too numerous to explain individually. However, techniques such as reframing, anchoring, triggering, matching, pacing and accessing cues should suffice to make the point.

Where methods of using NLP differ to the other methods of change is that they are more closely bound to harnessing the power of the unconscious mind to bring about change to benefit the individual. There is a feeling that the purpose is aimed at the satisfaction of the balance of an individual's self-interest

SUMMING UP
Imagination allows a suspension of the critical reality which is a fundamental aspect of hypnosis, active imagination, shamanism, and NLP. This allows an internal dialogue in symbolic, fantastic and metaphorical terms, so that a new reality is conceived, believed and therefore created. They all appear to be ways in which the unconscious mind and emotional reaction are accessed.

There are different representations of activities that occur in the unconscious mind, such as Jung's archetypes that seem to fit into the cultural background of the person involved. Shamanism has power animals, which, significantly always seem to fit into local environments rather than introducing locally unknown animals like polar bears in the Amazon and lions in Eskimo habitats. However, such representations occur very rarely in hypnosis, perhaps because there is no expectation of them, except when suggested.

The response at the heart of the four different approaches is assumed to be a human specific response which evokes the onset of theta waves, which signify a certain state of mind. The responses are too similar to psychotic responses, hallucinations etc. to be purely coincidental. Also psycho-active drugs produce a similar response, as experienced by anthropologists in older societies, and drug users in our society who seem to experience the belief that they can fly when using drugs such as LSD.

This response, and specifically the theta state, needs more research in order to establish the physiological/psychological connections. The symbolism and mythology involved seem to be part of the person's culture, therefore Jung was influenced by Greek and Egyptian mythology, whereas we are slightly lost in a more 'present day' society which has less emphasis on mythology except for Christianity, which is fading as an influence in a cross-cultural society, perhaps explaining the lack of symbolic figures encountered in hypnotherapy.

I believe that shamanism, active imagination, hypnosis and NLP rely on the same natural responses which allows thought to move from the unconscious mind into consciousness, and vice versa. This seems to be on a scale of reality-acceptance depending upon the belief system of the individual and the culture in which he lives, although psychotic episodes and hallucinogenic drug experiences also change the perception of reality. Whereas dreaming seems to be a natural 'leakage' of those unconscious thoughts, the four therapeutic methods are deliberate methods to elicit those thoughts and to expedite communication for, mostly, beneficial reasons.

The remaining question is how to best use other techniques within a culture which would broadly regard them as too bizarre to even contemplate. Perhaps this is the question that NLP answers, certainly in its approach to businesses that seem to accept a new approach when they would ordinarily regard hypnosis and hypnotherapy as a joke, thanks to stage hypnotists!

Self-Hypnosis

There is a question as to whether self-hypnosis is a special process that elicits an enchanted state of mind, or a way in which the imagination can be more readily accessed. The answer seems to be both, depending upon interpretation. The differences between self-hypnosis and applied hypnosis are, perhaps, more pertinent to the situation in which they are used.

Most applications of self-hypnosis are for relaxation and the use of imagination. For example, the escape from day-to-day life by imagining being in a 'special place' such as a sunny beach or by a magical waterfall allows the mind to dissociate from reality. This may be used for relaxation or to escape from the dentist's drill. It can be used to dissociate the mind from the body during childbirth.

Another use is for visualisation by, for example, athletes or by public speakers who mentally rehearse a brilliant performance. This can then translate into a better performance because the mind is less affected by negative thoughts that can inhibit the accomplishment of an objective. I believe that athletes, when they mentally rehearse, can benefit from something referred to as 'micro-twitch' in which the muscles work at a low level and as a result become strengthened.

This rehearsal, of course, may be done by applied hypnosis during an induction or as an outcome during hypnosis. Therefore, applied hypnosis to bring about the ability to relax when the client is in a specific situation may be seen as teaching self-hypnosis or as a 'post-hypnotic suggestion'.

Applications can be for dental phobics, sportsmen or women or for childbirth where the client is likely to need help when the therapist is unavailable or needs to work within her own private and intimate situation where the presence of a therapist is an intrusion.

So the difference appears to be in the application of hypnosis to imagine or visualise something that is desired against the use of hypnosis for the release of emotion in which case the mind needs to be kept focussed on issues that it would normally avoid.

The analogy that can be made is that of two bar magnets. Opposite poles attract so self-hypnosis can allow dreaming, visualising and can imagine positive outcomes because there is nothing to push the objective from the mind. For the analysis of emotional trauma it is as if like-poles repel each other and the outcome of joining them is difficult to achieve by the clients working by themselves.

It is hard to adhere to the belief that 'all hypnosis is self-hypnosis', therefore. Outside help is very necessary to achieve objectives that involve the release of thoughts that will close like a clam when the individual attempts to bring them to mind. A therapist will hold the shell open while the client extracts the memories that he/she is reluctant to expose to themselves or the therapist.

Metaphors

Metaphors are sessions in their own right. They capture the imagination by involving different senses to create a suitable environment, in the mind, for a positive outcome. The metaphor then gives a message for change in a creative way.

The therapist must have the ability to think laterally to sense the client's predicament as a story that can be told in figurative terms. We are raised in a world full of metaphors. As children we are told stories that have travelled through generations about dangers such as wandering into the woods on our own (Little Red Riding Hood), about the evilness of certain characters that we might meet (Monsters), about the possibilities of choking on apples (Sleeping Beauty) and so on.

We learn to count with beans because the logical concept of numbers is beyond a child. However, when foodstuffs are used, we gain a clearer picture of the notion at an early age because we can see beans but numbers are rational symbols that children have yet to learn to deal with.

That world never dies in adulthood; it is put away in a cupboard that can be opened by metaphors. We still have the ability to learn by example and those examples are stronger within the context of a story. When animals are used in those tales then the message seems to be more memorable, hence power animals in shamanism.

How often, as an adult, have you used any of the following?

She is a Wicked Witch.
A little bird told me.
He is a crafty fox.
Silly cow.
Snake in the grass.
The birds and the bees.
Dirty dog.

There are so many references to animals in our lives. We look for expressions that relate to behaviours that will give a better way to colour our speech.

When you construct a metaphor, look for analogy and the outcome that is needed. These two elements give direction.

You may have played the game;

'if I were a tree, I would be an oak because...'
'if I were a season, I would be summer because...'

This leads on to; 'if this client's problem is like an animal it would be a fine racehorse being used to transport rocks in panniers that were getting loaded to be more burdensome as life continues.'

This would represent a person who was being weighed down by the situation he/she was in and the burdens becoming greater with each passing day. The solution would be for the client to dump the problems and to start living a more enjoyable life as he/she was born to do. This might mean, in your metaphor, that the horse rears up, lets the panniers slide off his/her back and for the racehorse to be free of the ever increasing load.

This example, very condensed, is one that I took from one of my books of metaphors. When you write your own, let your imagination run free and then edit the story to ensure that it fits the client's needs.

A well constructed metaphor communicates with the client because it uses their imagination rather than logic to bring it into the context of their life. If a picture is worth a thousand words, then let your words create strong pictures that bring about positive changes.

This applies to goal setting as well as problem resolution. A well written metaphor can bring the best out of an athlete, a business person and everybody who needs to see a clear and clean future.

Analysis

I recommend analysis for every problem except for smoking (unless excessive), nail biting and weight control (if the excess weight is reasonably little).

Later in the book you will see in the treatment of specific problems that you will need to discover the root cause and deal with it. Analysis is the most effective way to do this.

Although some schools of thought believe that solutions to problems involve making a change in current, and therefore, future beliefs, I find it hard to build a new future on foundations made from sand. If a house is built on an old waste disposal dump and those gases and smells permeate the building it is pointless to fumigate and carry on as normal. The fumes will creep back. What is needed is to clear the debris from the dump and then clean the house.

In the same way, it is necessary to examine the past and to set a new basis for the lives of sufferers. We are dealing with emotion and they are timeless so they will continue to have an effect many years on, unless dealt with.

What is intended with analysis is the emotional recall of the client's life to openly remember events that have resulted in their problem. The introductory consultation enables you to gain information about the client's life and gives clues as to cause. These must be kept in your mind rather than leading to offering your theories. At this stage, the only input must be from the client. The Introductory Consultation should be about building trust as well as gaining information. Soon you will be told things that have been considered to be private and perhaps shameful beforehand.

The benefit of hypnosis is that it gives an apparent cloak of protection to the client within the sense of compliance with the therapist and therefore they will say whatever is in the mind because they feel that they will lose inhibitions and be able to stop fully censoring what they are revealing. Therefore the embarrassment that would be felt by saying those things in normal conversation is considerably diminished and therefore the subject matter of recall is allowed to come into the open.

During analysis you are going to act like a detective piecing together various bits of information. As the therapist you have two advantages over the client; namely you will write notes that you can refer back to and you will have an objective view about what is recalled. This adds the requirement that you need to be free of your own hang-ups. The process of analysis has to be gone through with any person who embarks on a career in therapy. Sometimes the client's recall could bring issues to the mind of the therapist that would be disturbing. Without clearing away those issues the therapist is in a weak and vulnerable position. (Also see Supervision.)

After an induction, ask the client to let their thoughts drift back through time and to recall, out loud, what they are thinking. Give your approval to the voicing of those thought without their editing. It makes no difference if those thoughts seem unimportant, irrelevant, shocking or embarrassing. In fact, if they are, so much the better.

I will say to a client, 'I have been doing this for X number of years, and there is nothing that I have not heard before'. Rather than boasting, this is to clear the path for the client to release any difficult memories or experiences that they might hold on to in front of a friend or relative who might bring them back to haunt the client in years to come.

The release of hitherto closely held memories is a process which I refer to as **mental vomiting**. As with bad food, it is better to get rid of it even if the process is painful and, seemingly, disgusting to the client. Jack-in-a-box memories pop-up when the client trusts you enough to let them go. Rather than mistaking these as repressed memories that force themselves into consciousness, this is the client allowing suppressed thoughts to emerge. The idea of repression, I feel, is a fallacy. The client has never found anybody that they trusted enough

39

to relate the memory to. If you consider that Freud wrote in German and you look up a translation for repression and suppression, you will see that they both translate to German as the same word, Unterdrückung. Do we misunderstand his meaning because of a translation error?

Catharsis or abreaction is the release of tightly held memories when the client feels safe to do so. The screaming and highly emotional letting go that is portrayed in films or on TV can happen but when the client lets go as if pressing the valve on a pressure cooker, the explosion that happens when the lid is taken off suddenly is controlled.

There is no point in repressing something, with the mind's theoretical aim of obliterating it, only for it to influence behaviour and then explode into consciousness. The mind suppressing a memory is a better idea.

The therapist needs to be quiet and non-judgemental during this process. If the client is slow to start or reports having no thoughts, then you can ask "what is your earliest memory?" We all have one. This places the client into a new time frame from which their recall can proceed without the therapist asking leading questions, which should always be avoided, or deliberately stirring up associations.

What you are leading up to by asking for recall is the client's arrival at an event, or series of events, considered to be traumatic. You are waiting for those events that caused an emotional reaction of fear, revulsion, shame or self-judgement. It is the emotion that you are seeking.

As will be explained later, emotional memories are stored in a part of the brain called the amygdala which triggers the fight-or-flight response when something considered to be threatening or dangerous occurs. When a like situation is perceived then the alarm bells ring, the client goes into a red alert state to avoid the damage from that earlier situation from happening again. The brain can bring back all sorts of associated smells, sounds, sights and physical effects with those traumatic memories. The thing that is missing, to protect us, is a sense of dilution of fear through time. In our primeval history, a puff-adder would be as dangerous to an old man as it was to the same person as a child. Survival means that we should respond in the same way to a threat at any point in our lives.

However, when the reaction is inappropriate, then the client suffers from the negative effect of the emotion in many different ways.

The amygdala, although there are two, has to learn that the reaction to the original trigger and like situations can be ameliorated by giving a different outcome so that it can view the situation(s) with calmness and control.

Real experiences, and imagined ones, of trauma or frightening incidents, will set down reactions that help to avoid those dangers if those circumstances arise again.

This is protective if similar events are dangerous, but if they are safe then the reaction is inappropriate, unsuitable and debilitating. By encouraging the client to recall the details and emotions of the original event and modifying the outcome to an acceptable or beneficial outcome, then a new calm reaction in those situations will occur.

So how is this done in detail?

If you are an analytical therapist, then I feel you should take a part in the analysis of the client. In other words, rather than sitting session after session waiting for the abreaction or catharsis (the sudden release of emotion by recall), you should be able to gently point the client in the direction of letting go.

Rather than blurting out your theories, the process has to be gentle. But waiting for twelve sessions before contributing any information is postponing the resolution and increasing the client's cost dramatically. You should have a good idea of cause after three or four sessions. So should the client.

The final realisation of the cause for the client can happen by the therapist using analogy or metaphor, sometimes by encouraging the client to revisit disclosed experiences.

The purpose of analysis is to expose the original event and how it affected the client. Then it is necessary to move onto a different, positive, outcome. For example, a flying phobic should come to enjoy flying rather than just coping. Or somebody who has been sexually abused should be able to expect love, tenderness and respect from their current, innocent, partner thereby allowing sexual activity rather than countering with fear, disdain or frigidity. To do this they must be aware of why they were unable to enjoy the experiences in the first place.

In the twenty-first century we, and our clients, have different attitudes to those that Freud would have encountered. We must bring our approach to analysis up to date if we are to offer efficient and effective therapy. We should never expect to keep our clients in a vacuum of treatment that is waiting for an admission to a therapist of something that is known already but has been unsaid by either party. If you call yourself an analyst, what are you analysing?

Our role is to facilitate the appeasement of the symptoms of the problem and to bring about relief. Our role should never be a chaperone to secrets that are known to the client but not confessed until the client has had enough repetitive treatment to frustrate them to the extent that they feel they can only bring therapy to an end by releasing something that they have been aware of all along.

After a number of sessions you can help by asking for clarification of some of the recall during sessions. This throws a broad focus at the client without suggesting that you have found the cause. Detail should be kept to a minimum. Again you should ask a non-specific question, an open question, and listen to the response. Make notes as you do so.

A note of caution. Playing the smart detective, knowing who-done-it from the beginning and then finding the proof might have worked for Columbo but you have to be neutral and allow the client to name the cause.

You must keep an open mind until you are sure. If you jump to conclusions and act too soon with the clients, then you run the risk of making them go into denial, even if you got it right. Resolution is a subtle process.

ORIGINAL TRAUMA.
A situation or event is seen as real threat and causes fear.

SIMILAR EVENTS TO THE ORIGINAL TRAUMA CAUSE NEW PROBLEMS.
For example a spider phobic panicking at the sight of the top of a tomato or a snake phobic panicking when seeing a hose pipe.

AN EMOTIONAL CHANGE BECAUSE A NEW OUTCOME OR ASSOCIATION IS PERCEIVED OR MADE.
e.g. spiders seen as allies in the fight against flies and mosquitoes

MODIFIED OUTCOME WITH NO DEBILITATING REACTION.
When the client can sense that the sense of threat has gone in the current and future time frames and can be free from the old problem.

The above diagram shows that when the mind is reminded of the original trauma then the original response can follow. When the outcome is modified, then similar stimuli may be disregarded. Even with this change of reaction, safety will still always be evaluated. A person released from an irrational fear of heights will still avoid standing at the edge of a cliff.

PART THREE

Information for the Therapist

The following section contains information that therapists should be aware of. Some of it is essential and some is for consideration.

Supervision

A breakdown truck that breaks down on its way to fix your car never bodes well for the quality of service that you will get.

It almost goes without saying that the therapist is vulnerable. Apart from losing your own problems through analysis when you are training it is vital that you have a 'supervisor'. This is somebody who will offer help, wisdom and an ear to hear any issues that you might develop as a therapist.

We can be affected by the problems of the world as well as those of our clients. Unless taken care of as we go along, these can lead to something called 'therapist burn-out.' This is a dramatic term for a dramatic outcome.

As tough, stoic and macho as we think we might be, there are darts than can slip through chinks in our armour if we have them. Even then, we never know where the chinks are unless we feel a twinge at an unexpected moment.

You need a supervisor for your health rather than to keep an association happy because they require that you have one.

Associations will put you in touch with a supervisor if you are looking. They want mentally healthy therapists on their books rather than gibbering wrecks.

The term supervisor or supervision is in a way misleading. Rather than being a supervisor as in a line-manager, the role is that of a consultant or advisor. The purpose is to keep your mind clean and to be able to offer different perspectives on the treatments that you are offering to your clients.

Human Lives

**The most perfect thing about humans is our lack of perfection.
That attribute has driven us to search for better answers.**

Human beings are animals who can think and speak to each other, although we have a multitude of languages from nation to nation. We are no different to other creatures apart from having a more sophisticated language and an advanced ability to use tools.

Where we differ from other animals is that we live in crowded conditions where we hunt for money. We still gather, but from safe locations such as supermarkets. We have rules and laws that set behaviour standards. We have a sense of conscience that is given to us by authority figures and it tells us internally, as well as externally, what we should do or avoid doing, and that if we do something that is prohibited then we should feel guilty, whatever that means.

What we have in common with all creatures is a hard-wiring that drives us to certain courses of action. These fitted beautifully into the primeval human who was weak bodied and lacked the ability to run as fast as most predators.

This makes understanding of problems easier to find. To assume that we are highly sophisticated creations, remote from other animals, makes us look for the flaws in our civilised nature rather than to see those primal behaviours as the ones we are struggling to control.

Now, we have weapons that make us dominant and we have safe shelters from every other predator and pest. We have moved our bodies into those places and we have moved our conscious thoughts with them. What still haunts us now that we are 'civilised' is that set of old cave-dweller instincts and reactions.

We are basically primeval creatures with a very, very thin veneer of what we call civilisation. Under that brittle surface we are driven by basic survival motivations; namely safety, sex, gratification and greed. The nature of humans is that we are old pack animals dressed in modern clothing.

We go into tribal battles, but now in football grounds. We go to War as mega tribes. We still live in packs although we live as small individual units, families, or as individuals on our own. We still protect our territories and possessions with violence, if necessary.

On holiday we strip ourselves on beaches to be as naked as cave dwellers, or we wallow around watering holes, known as swimming pools. We still sleep upstairs to keep ourselves safe from predators at night, although we live in rooms during the day that offer a more restricted view of the neighbourhood. Despite being potentially dangerous, we all enjoy log fires in our lounges. We enjoy cooking over open fires such as barbeques. And so on.

Yet, in our modern lives, we can isolate ourselves to the point of loneliness. We can live far away from our kinsfolk. That rarely happened 50,000 years ago. We have set up the very conditions that we struggle with. We have created emotional conflicts that battle with the modern urge to be logical.

Children behave as our very old ancestors did because they struggle to understand the rules of logic. They can often show themselves to be the sweet faced primitive creatures that live within all of us, but we also know that they have the capacity to be very cruel.

Freud and Jung assumed that the human psyche is a victim of conflict between the unconscious and somewhat 'primitive' drives and conscious desires. They were right in that respect.

When treating clients our task, as therapists, is to reconcile the instinctual behaviour with the way in which our lives now unfold and with the resultant pressures and strife. Rather than being wolves in sheep's clothing, we are apes in designer clothes.

Previous Lives

The term that confuses therapists and clients alike is 'regression'. For clients it usually means past or previous lives and to the therapist analytical regression to an earlier stage of life.

I have attended conferences where therapists have boasted that "85% of my clients will spontaneously slip into a previous life!" Well, all I can say is that after seeing thousands of clients over a great number of years, I am still waiting for my first spontaneous previous life client! Either I am doing something wrong or the other "past-life" therapists are making leading suggestions that precipitate the notion of an existence before this life.

What results is the client's ability to blame their problems onto somebody else rather than to face up to what has happened in their own lifetime. Certainly, issues can be addressed vicariously, but the resolution of a problem has to be with the person in front of you rather than with their imaginary friend, or enemy.

Please believe me; the only previous lives in our minds are the primeval drivers that make us act in an emotional way and that contradict our modern rational needs. This is the hard-wiring that we would call instincts in non-human animals, the ability to build bird-nests or for baby creatures to find teats for milk from the mother.

As a serious point, past-life therapy, unless it can be proved to be based on hard evidence makes a mockery of therapy. Clients arrive with problems and the treatment, as if dealing with a ghost that haunts, can do nothing other than harm. People's problems occur from events in their earlier lives, as they exist now. That is where the cause and effects have come from. To blame problems on a previous life misdemeanour relegates the cause to something beyond what a professional therapist can, or should, deal with.

We should never be spiritualists calling upon departed souls for forgiveness or responsibility for blame, we have to deal with what is real.

Having said all of the above, the most serious side to previous lives is that the therapist is almost replicating the signs and symptoms of paranoid schizophrenia. These signs are delusions and hallucinations. It is thought that between 1% and 3% of the population will, at some time suffer from paranoid schizophrenia. Does a previous/past life therapist know what they are risking with their clients? Is there a possibility that such a problem could be created or exacerbated? We deal with neurotics rather than with psychotics.

If you want to be a therapist you should be knowledgeable about what is referred to as 'Abnormal Psychology'.

Another issue is that of 'false memory syndrome'. As careful as a therapist might be in avoiding the creation of memories of sexual abuse that are untrue, it strikes me as strange that the creation of a previous life that can never be substantiated falls into the same trap.

A therapist who can lead clients into believing that they have lived before by 'leading' them must be at risk of getting clients to falsely think that they have been abused.

How can we dismiss one thing whilst accepting the same thing with a different name?

OK!
Would you like a previous life?

It is easy. Answer the following <u>leading</u> questions:
- Think of an era two lifetimes ago (i.e. roughly 140 years ago, say 1870)
- Where are you in the World?
- Are you male or female?

- Do you live in the country, town or city?
- Are you young, middle-aged or old?
- Are you married?
- Do you have children?
- What do you do as an occupation?
- Look in a mirror and smile. How you look?
- How did you die?
- What is your first name?
- What is your surname?
- What is your date of birth?
- What are your siblings called?
- What are your parent's names?

You will now have a mental picture of a person. This comes from nothing more than your imagination. You will have noticed that it gets progressively harder to answer questions as they need you to find more information from your mind. Things that would be known spontaneously make you think. Your memory is tested as you need to find a time and place that you have some ideas about. Think back to your image in the mirror.

You looked like a 21st century person. You had good teeth, well groomed hair and you were clean. Now consider dental hygiene, hair care, bathing arrangements and sanitary care in that era. Do you still believe in previous lives?

With leading questions, put cunningly, you can create the notion of a previous life or lots of them with some people. With a bit more imagination you can even create the idea of a future life.

I think that previous lives are nothing more than a dangerous party game.

The Brain and Therapy

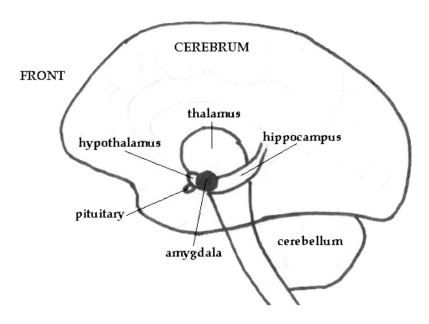

The brain is the seat of logic AND emotion. We grow up in a World that rates logic as a higher attribute than emotion but as therapists, we are most often dealing with our clients' helplessness in framing disturbing life experiences in their correct way.

As therapists we need to understand the way the brain/mind works in order to find a better way through the emotional fog in which our clients live. The following will never teach you to become a brain surgeon but it will give better understanding of some of the processes that control the symptoms that you will meet. It is simplified to show relevance to therapy rather than being an exposition of brain physiology.

If you want more detailed descriptions of the parts of the brain, then I would refer you to the Internet or to books that fully explain current ideas. These seem to change and a lot of information is based on monkey or rat brains!

THE LIMBIC SYSTEM

The limbic system is a collection of structures including the hippocampus, amygdala, anterior thalamic nuclei, and limbic cortex, which have a direct influence on aspects of emotion, behaviour, long term memory, and smell. "Smell memory" is an important part of emotion. We can sense the aroma of after-shaves and perfumes long after we first experienced them. I can still recall the smell that my children had after they were born in much the same way as a mother sheep must recognize the lambs that are hers!

The following are considered to be part of the limbic system:

Amygdala
There are, in fact, two amygdalas. Each one is about the size of an almond. They are referred to as the storage part of the brain for emotional trauma as they set off the fight-or-flight response when a danger is perceived. This is a powerful trigger even when a situation is a similar or imagined event. What the amygdala misses is an awareness of time and the means to critically evaluate the way it responds. The events that happened many years ago are as fresh as if they happened today.

Part of therapy is to change the outcome of an event so that a positive ending is now stored. This involves reliving the event and all its emotional content **but** when the client is able to be relaxed and able to experience different emotional responses so a new consequence may be elicited that is more controlled and less alarming.

Hippocampus
Sitting next to the amygdalas are the hippocampi, from the Greek hippo for horse and kampo for sea monster. These are two long and convoluted structures, a bit like a seahorse in shape in the human brain, that have a role in the formation of new memories and spatial awareness.

Hypothalamus
In relation to the rest of the brain, and to its functions, the

hypothalamus is extremely small, roughly the size of a walnut. Its name is to do with its relative location to the thalamus, (hypo- is ancient Greek for 'under'), rather than to its functional relationship to the thalamus. The role ascribed to it is 'homeostasis', the preservation of the state of the body in a balanced way. However it contributes far more than just a steady state.

The hypothalamus works mostly by negative feedback. That is, low levels of a hormone in the blood supplying the hypothalamus stimulate the release of a hormone which in turn stimulates the pituitary, which in turn stimulates the target gland to secrete the hormone until the level rises to the point where it inhibits the releasing hormone by the hypothalamus.

It is possible to summarise the main functions of the hypothalamus as follow:

(1) Endocrine Control
The pituitary gland is the master of the endocrine system that controls the secretions of hormones from a variety of other glands that enable the body to maintain a 'steady state', or 'homeostasis'. The pituitary is actually controlled by the hypothalamus.

(2) Neurosecretion
The hypothalamus produces the hormone oxytocin, which promotes contractions in childbirth and in stimulating the nipples for breastfeeding along with prolactin which stimulates milk production. It is also has a role in social behaviours such as bonding. Sometimes mothers will produce milk in the presence of children that are not hers.

It also releases hormones connected to the maturation of ova (females) and the production of sperm in males.

It produces antidiuretic hormone (ADH) which controls levels of urine production by affecting the levels of re-absorption of water by the kidneys. It also monitors water balance and stimulates thirst or drinking.

(3) Autonomic Nervous System (ANS)
Autonomic derives from autonomous, meaning that there is no conscious control. This is divided into two branches; the sympathetic and the parasympathetic. The sympathetic branch is responsible for the 'fight-or-flight' response and the parasympathetic for countering it and for relaxation.

(4) Temperature
It also regulates the balance of the operating requirements of the body such as temperature through thermoreceptors that gain information from blood that circulates through it. It controls body temperature through the Autonomic Nervous System. The mechanisms for temperature control include sweating and panting to reduce it, and shivering to raise it.

(5) Food and Water Intake
In addition, its actions have an effect on overt behaviour as well as internal balancing procedures. These include hunger by monitoring chemical balance and the amount of nutrients in the blood. It can determine the commencement and termination of eating. Leptin is a protein that is produced by fat cells when people overeat. The hypothalamus detects leptin levels in the blood and, if they are high, it will decrease appetite.

(6) Biological Clocks
It is also responsible for the maintenance of biological clocks or circadian rhythms, involving other parts of the endocrine system, for example, the pineal gland which monitors light and secretes the hormone melatonin which affects sleep patterns.

(7) Emotional Reactions
These include: fear, rage, aversion pleasure and reward. To quote Gray's Anatomy, "The emotional content of an individual consists of two main elements: the *subjective feeling state* or *affective tone*, and the *objective physical accompaniments* which constitute *emotional expression*. For the full integration of both these aspects of emotion, with changes in the internal and external environment, and with other cerebral

activities, the essential neurological structures are an intact hypothalamus, limbic system, and pre-frontal cortex."

One of the striking things about the hypothalamus is its connection between major physiological functions and the emotions, which appear to have a chemical basis in hormones. Some hormones are associated with the emotions of the 'fight or flight' reaction, including fear and some pleasure, physical and sexual.

The hypothalamus produces corticotrophin-releasing hormone which stimulates the pituitary gland to produce adrenocorticotrophic hormone (ACTH) which stimulates the adrenal glands to produce steroids which promote muscle development. ACTH also stimulates the liver to release stored sugars. Interestingly it has a relationship to stress resistance in the immediate 'fight or flight' response. However in the longer term, secretion of ACTH has less desirable effects such as the lowering of the immune response and increase in blood pressure, amongst others. Therefore stress disturbs homeostasis.

The Limbic Cortex
This has a relevance to judgement, insight, motivation and mood. It is also involved in emotional responses. It is affected by alcohol and accounts for loss of judgement by heavy drinkers. It also effects mood and has a relationship with depression.

Smell, olfaction, in this part of the brain can cause emotional responses through its connection with the amygdala and hypothalamus.

The Thalamus
The thalamus is, in fact two egg-shaped masses of nerve cells and fibres which are joined. They are located near the centre of the brain. These thalami will be referred to in the singular as appears to be convention. Relevant to the limbic system are the anterior thalamic nuclei which have a relation to alertness, learning and memory

The thalamus has three main functions:

(1) Receiving and processing sensory information, and transmitting that information to the cerebral cortex. Most sensory receptors pass the information they receive to the thalamus as electrical impulses. The exception is olfactory information (smell), which is passed directly to the limbic system. It has been suggested that the thalamus conducted sorting of sensory information in the 'old brain', which would account for it being an important part of the current route to the more advanced 'modern brain', the cerebrum.

(2) Passing information about complex motor actions to the cerebellum. (The cerebellum is involved in maintaining physical balance and for coordinating muscular movements in order to ensure smoothness of action.)

(3) Some sleep and waking functions. In rapid eye movement sleep (REM), information travels from the pons (the bridge between the medulla, the first structure that emerges from the spinal cord and the midbrain) to the visual cortex.

Summary and conclusions
The brain is complex and the above is a brief description of some of the parts that control and mediate the emotional responses with which therapists work. How they function gives insight rather than a methodology.

The processes of therapy have to have a base of knowledge, however, in order to avoid falling into strange beliefs about how we achieve results. We need to fight fire with fire. The best way to change negative emotional response is by creating positive ones in the parts of the brain that contain them.

We are much longer lived than we would have been 50,000 years ago and we have fallen victim to the battle between logic and emotion. In order to live stress reduced lives we must be able to, once in a while, set logic to one side and let our emotional burdens become emotional blessings.

The reactions of our ancestors, stored in our modern minds are far less relevant to 21st century life. However the responses of anger, fear, hunger and the rest still play key roles in our lives.

Whereas our ancestors were contained by the environment, we have more freedom and opportunity to express those emotions and feelings, yet that freedom, ironically, allows them to rule us at times.

We as therapists, have to help our clients, and ourselves, to come to terms with the problems caused by our nature.

Environmental or Genetic Influences?

There are many different influences in life that can influence behaviours and attitudes. The argument as to whether these are nature or nurture should never be seen as two polar extremes. Both can have effects, there can be a cocktail. As therapists we are unable to change genetic influences, but we can change behaviours. Sometimes the idea of a problem being genetic is a cop-out. Please consider the following:

Excess weight
If a person grows up in a household where there is a culture of excessive and unhealthy eating, perhaps that person becomes fat because it is an expectation rather than a genetic dispensation. There are other factors in obesity, but more of that later. The escape, for the client, is a realisation that changes in their attitude towards food can make an enormous difference. The client's parents would have lacked a quality of life and that should be a huge incentive for the client to lose weight by eating a healthy diet and taking more exercise. As mentioned, factors involved in obesity are many and you should read the chapter on weight control.

Depression
As with weight, home influences can make a difference with depression. A child or young person growing up in a household that lacks cheer, where everything is seen through a cloud of gloom, is likely to be unable to see a brighter side of life when he/she grows up. A depressed person needs to be able to look to a bright and cheery future. The glass must be seen as half full rather than half empty.

Smoking
Again parental behaviour can give a child a false sense of 'cool' things to do. With smoking, peer pressure also plays a monumental part, but when a smoker reaches an age when he/she can make their own decisions on 'cool' or 'idiotic' things to do, they are more ready to quit the deadly activity.

The Human Psyche According to Freud and Jung

**What the founders of psycho-analysis really thought.
Do we take the men too seriously and should we
question the modern relevance of their theories ?**

This part is added as there is confusion about what the two men developed as therapy and its relevance to modern times. The important thing to remember is that their era was very different to current times. Now, clients are more open, less ashamed and will talk more freely about their problems.

Perhaps Freud was obsessed by sex and Jung seen as an eccentric but their methods should be seen as the starting point rather than the definitive way to conduct therapy. Some aspects are very relevant today such as Jung's active imagination, but we must, perhaps, move on.

The models of both men assume that the human psyche is a victim of conflict between the unconscious and somewhat primitive drives and conscious desires. There is a fundamental motivational force, libido, which represents those inner drives and seeks fulfilment. These inner desires are thought to be present at birth, and as the human grows, conflict arises in their expression in a world which does not allow those drives to be fully expressed because there are external controls and pressures. The structures of the mind are stated as if they were distinct and identifiable parts, each with an assumed role to play. Obviously their theories are models of the mind rather than attempts to explain precise areas as an anatomical study would do. Both Freud and Jung were essentialists, they explained phenomena in terms of essences, the assumed forces underlying the causes of behaviour rather than studying the phenomena themselves.

The following will outline the theoretical models of the mind proposed by Freud and Jung.

FREUD

Initially, Freud identified two parts of the mind, the conscious and the unconscious. He later proposed that the mind consisted of three main parts, the 'id', the 'ego' and the 'super-ego', although he also proposed other subsidiary parts such as the 'unconscious ego' and the 'pre-conscious'. I have taken the model which Freud defined in 1923 and which includes his revisions.

The conscious mind is the part that we are aware of. It is the link between the external world and the inner, unconscious systems. Freud later described it as the ego. The ego represents consciousness, and uses the secondary thinking process of reason, common sense and the power to delay immediate response. It is derived from the 'id', developing as a result of stimuli from the external world impinging upon the senses. The ego is an intermediary between the 'id' and the external world. Its prime function is self-preservation.

Put very simplistically, the unconscious, later the 'id', is that part of the mind that is not the conscious. Freud's early model was that the unconscious was derived from repression, and it therefore consisted of impulses, thoughts and feelings which were unacceptable to the conscious ego.

Repression is defined as the conflict of instinct with the ego, the disowning of emotion, the process that removes unpleasant thoughts from the conscious mind. Although Freud assumed that the unconscious is the home of repression, he made the qualification that repression is only part of the unconscious. Later in his life he changed his concept of the unconscious to the *agency instituting repression derived from the ego, the conscious part*. Resistance is the force which institutes repression and maintains it. This implies that part of the ego is unconscious, the unconscious ego.

The preconscious is a 'holding area'. When thoughts (psychical acts) pass from the unconscious to the conscious they are transferred via the preconscious from which those thoughts can become conscious without resistance when the right conditions apply. Those thoughts are not repressed.

Freud originally postulated that neuroses arose as a result of conflict between the unconscious and the conscious. He later amended this to neurosis being *'the antithesis between coherent ego and the repressed which is split off from it'*. However, *'it is still true that all that is repressed is unconscious, but not all that is unconscious is repressed...A part of the ego...undoubtedly is unconscious...and is not latent like the preconscious'*. This is the part of the mind that he called the unconscious ego.

Freud described the id as the primitive part of the mind, which contains the inherited characteristics and instincts. It uses primary thought processes, those of condensation, displacement, symbolism, hallucinatory wish-fulfilment as dreams. It ignores concepts of time and space, and contrasts such as light and darkness, high and deep by considering them as identical. It is governed by basic mental dynamics, including the avoidance of 'unpleasure' caused by instinctual tension. This, it is assumed, can only be done by the achievement of the satisfaction of instinctual needs which are accompanied by pleasure. This is the 'pleasure principle'.

The 'reality principle' is similar in concept to the pleasure principle, but it involves deriving instinctual gratification by accommodating information and objects which relate to the external world, therefore it is related to the ego.

The 'super-ego' is the part of the ego in which self-observation and self criticism develop. The super-ego is an agency which prolongs parental authority, a third force. It traces to back to narcissism.

As the child acquires cultural and ethical ideas, libidinal impulses undergo repression, and the child cannot achieve its ideal-self, its standard of perfection, the ego-ideal, that to which its own ego does not conform. The super-ego watches, and becomes the parental standards of prohibition and criticism, and, subsequently, standards of society. It therefore becomes an instrument of guilt.

JUNG

For Jung, the psyche is the mind in totality. Its function is to maintain balance between opposing forces. Jung's conception of the psyche is of a system which is dynamic, in constant movement, and at the same time self-regulating; he calls the general psychic energy libido, but his concept of libido is more expansive than that of Freud.

Like Freud, Jung identified the conscious and the unconscious, but he described them in different developmental ways by defining two types of unconscious mind.

Jung considered the conscious aspect of the psyche like an island rising from the sea. The island is the ego, the knowing, willing 'I', the centre of consciousness. Like Freud's belief that the ego develops from the id, Jung believed that the conscious...'*grows out of an unconscious psyche which is older than it, and which goes on functioning together with it or even in spite of it'*.

Jung believed that the conscious can forget, repress what it does not like, or what is not socially acceptable. Repression, for Jung, means an almost deliberate withdrawal of attention so that the thing which is to be repressed is expelled from consciousness. The part which stretches between the ego and the unconscious, which contains subliminal perceptions, repressed or forgotten memories is the personal unconscious, as distinct from the collective unconscious, the home of instincts and archetypes. Both the personal and the collective unconscious are the submerged parts, those under the sea.

The 'shadow' is found in the personal unconscious. It comes close to Freud's id in that it is the part that it primitive and base in nature. It is the pure instinctive man. The personal unconscious does not fully correspond to Freud's id, however. It is the personal part of the id, the part that is the result of individuality, the part that is added to the far greater part of the unconscious, the collective unconscious. Not only is it personal, however, it is also collective. Jung believed that there was a common root of instincts and behaviours which are species typical.

These instincts and archetypes are present in the collective unconscious, the part of the mind which is a common feature of all mankind, not connected in a spiritual of telepathic way, but having stemmed from a common genetic source.

The force which represses thoughts into the shadow derives from the 'moral complex'. The moral complex is an archetype that contains the drive to conform to the values of the society of the individual.

The opposing, collective aspect to the shadow is the 'persona'. The repression of the 'shadow' tendencies, drives or instincts leads to a conflict between the true nature of an individual and the role he plays in society. This compromise results in the individual projecting characteristics which are adopted rather than natural. This adoption of a role, the persona, is a collective phenomenon.

The clash between the shadow and the persona exemplifies the underlying principle of psychodynamic psychology, that of conflict between opposing forces. However Jung emphasised more than Freud did that the clash was to achieve balance rather than create disharmony. The opposites were also different in sort, Freud's being things like love and hate, innate drives, whereas Jung's opposites were within the structure of the mind. For example, Jung ascribed a feminine side to a man, the 'anima' and a masculine side to a woman, the 'animus'. The anima of a man represents the image of the man/woman relationship and is, at first, generalised. It later becomes conscious and modified through real experience of women, the first experience being that of his relationship with his mother.

This closely touches Freud's development of the Oedipus complex but in Freud's view the mother becomes an object for libidinal impulses rather than being a personification of the image of the archetype and thus a model for attitudes to women. Jung applies the same logic in the way the animus relates to the development of women. However Jung attributed different qualities to the anima and the animus, the anima producing moods, and the animus producing opinions. In this way they are mediators between the conscious and the unconscious mind.

65

Another archetype is the 'old wise man' which represents intelligence, knowledge and insight. This is the part of the mind that can silently advise, the part which gives answers to problems in dreams or in a creative insight. The female equivalent is 'the great mother', but with more pronounced 'feminine' traits of love, understanding and self-sacrifice. (This is certainly not the archetype of modern feminism!) The archetypes are voices of authority, although not equivalent to Freud's super-ego.

The most metaphysical archetype is that of 'the self'. The self exemplifies the reconciliation of all the inner conflicts, the achievement of balance and the goal towards which man should move if he is to achieve peace. It is the representation of God as a concept rather than as a creation of the church.

INSTINCTS

Freud had a changing view of instincts. He thought of instincts as an internal driving force. He initially identified two prime instincts, self-preservation, pertaining to ego and the sexual instinct, pertaining to the 'object'. He later added the death instinct, perhaps because he had an extremely pessimistic view of death, as he got closer to his own.

The aggression instinct, derived from the death instinct, was added in 1915 in 'Instincts and their Vicissitudes'. Freud recognises the 'aggressive instinct' as a constituent of the ego distinct from the sexual instinct. This was fully acknowledged in 'Beyond the Pleasure Principle' in 1920. In The Pleasure Principle, Freud's concern was with the avoidance of pain rather than the pursuit of pleasure. The pleasure principle and wish fulfilment govern the id's primary thought process; it represents the inner desire to achieve what is desired by instinctive nature.

Jung took a much broader view of instincts, although still recognising them as a driving force. He placed them in the collective unconscious. *'What we properly call instincts are physiological urges, and are perceived by the senses. But at the same time, they also manifest themselves in fantasies and often reveal their presence only by symbolic images. These manifestations are what I call the archetypes.'* (Jung. Man and his Symbols.)

LIBIDO

Both men called the force deriving from the instincts as libido. Libido is assumed to be a form of mental energy. *'We have defined the concept of libido as a quantitatively variable force which could serve as a measure of processes and transformations occurring in the field of sexual excitation.'* (Freud, 1915). Freud further differentiates sexual libido from other 'psychical energy'. He perceived libido as the major instinctive force. Freud defined the quantity of energy attached to an object representation or mental structure as cathexis.

Jung thought that *'the concept of libido must not be thought of as implying a force as such, any more than does the concept of energy in physics; it is simply a convenient way of describing the observed phenomena.'* Jung assumed that libido flows between two opposites; pairs of opposites being fundamental to most of Jung's theories. Jung called the forward flow of libido progression, the active adaptation to the environment; whereas the backwards flow, regression, was an adaptation to inner needs. The comparison is thus with a liquid, which over-stretches the analogy perhaps, although it asserts its dynamic nature. On one hand libido is considered not to be a force, but there is a contradictory assertion that the libido will 'leak', 'burst dams' and 'flood'.

Whereas Freud concentrated his theories on the early childhood stages of life, Jung considered that development was an ongoing process, one that took a different direction after mid-life.

The overwhelming motivational force in life, according to Freud is the sexual drive, or libido. Freud distinguished three main phases of childhood sexual development. He argued that different areas of the body formed the main focus for the expression of sexual libido, and that those areas became attached to an external object. 'Object' is used here as a thing, or person, outside the individual. Freud uses the term 'pregenital' to describe phases in which the genitals are presumed to have not taken their role as 'erotogenic zones' and other objects become areas of sexual focus in which the child derives 'auto-erotic' satisfaction. Freud's belief was that neurotic symptoms developed as a result of the repression of the sexual impulses in childhood.

My **personal** opinion is that men are fascinated by women's breasts because they are hidden and to see and touch them is an intimate thing when we are sexually mature. To a child a breast is a food source and little more. When we compare Western women to those in tribes in Africa and South America where exposed breasts are the norm, there are no strange theories about children having erotic fantasies about their mothers!

Freud initially identified the first two phases described below, and later added a third.

The 'oral' phase lasts up to the end of the first year. As the name suggests, the child's world is primarily perceived through contact with the mouth. Freud called this phase the 'cannibalistic pregenital sexual organisation', during which sexual activity has not been differentiated from the consumption of food. Freud makes the assumption that the breast is perceived both as a sexual object and an object for the provision of food. The sexual activity, he asserts, continues later in life as other oral activities such as thumb sucking.

The phase which occurs in the second and third years of the child's life is the 'sadistic-anal phase', so called by Freud but more usually referred to as the anal, or anal-sadistic phase. During this stage, the child develops a concept of bodily control including locomotion, bodily and manual activity. He also develops control of defecation, the mastery of which is the active sexual focus, and the erotogenic mucous membrane of the anus the centre of passive sexual activity. This is the point at which starts to differentiate power and control as that of his own and that of his parents.

The 'phallic' phase happens at about four or five years of age and it is when a child realises that the real source of sexual pleasure is seated in the genitals and is exhibited by childhood masturbation. At this point the Oedipus complex assumes that every boy develops a sexual interest in his mother, and therefore develops hostile feelings towards his father. This is a conflict that has to be resolved. The male child develops the castration complex, a fear of castration by his father as a punishment. He further proposed that the sexual feelings of the child toward the mother were switched over to other women as a reaction to the threat of castration resulting from hostile feelings from the father. Therefore the resolution of the complex is the identification with the parent of the same sex.

Freud developed the concept of his Oedipus theory from his own self-analysis and assumed the principle to be universal. He traced his feelings back to seeing his mother naked whilst on a train journey when he was very young.

Jung did not define stages of development in distinct time bands. His concept of development was the acquisition of the different archetypes as the person grew. However he did differentiate between early years and later years in terms of needs. In the early years up to the mid-life point (35-40 years), the main need is that of material and intellectual acquisition, and self establishment in society. The second stage is that of reconciliation and fulfilment. This becomes the drive towards 'individuation'.

Both Freud and Jung proposed that the root of neurotic behaviour was in the conflict concerning the instincts.

Freud's view was that the conflict was with the ego and instincts, and Jung said, *'What we call civilised consciousness has steadily separated itself from the basic instincts. But these instincts have not disappeared. They have merely lost their contact with our consciousness and are thus forced to assert themselves in an indirect fashion. This may be by means of physical symptoms in the case of a neurosis, or by means of incidents of various kinds, like unaccountable moods, unexpected forgetfulness, or mistakes in speech.'* (Jung. Man and his Symbols).

As in other issues, Jung applied a positive and optimistic view. *'Every neurosis has an aim; it is an attempt to compensate for a one-sided attitude to life, and a voice, as it were, drawing attention to a side of personality that has been neglected or repressed'.*

Freud's theory of the human psyche is one based on internal conflict.

The repression of the affect produces neurotic symptoms because it cannot be discharged. Repression is the conflict of instinct with ego.

Freud claimed that disowned affect gives rise to physical symptoms in the case of hysteria. The disowning of affect is the process of repression, the first defence mechanism, the process of banishing unpleasant thoughts and memories from the conscious mind. Freud concluded that the disowned affect gave rise to neurotic symptoms. It was initially assumed to be primarily connected to trauma. In addition to external trauma, however, Freud also included instinctual impulses. The emotions involved are shameful, painful or frightening. Freud asserted that trauma could be traced back to a pre-dating original trauma of a sexual kind.

He assumed that the early sexual experiences resulted from seduction, an idea which he later modified to one of childhood fantasy. He felt that the frequency of seduction, or abuse that would have been necessary to account for so many hysterics was not believable. He also would not accept that as some of his siblings suffered hysterical symptoms, his father would have to be implicated in their seduction in order to account for that to have happened. By his self-reflection, he was aware of his own childhood fantasies. He also identified a group of neuroses caused by sexual impulses which had not been discharged; for example, masturbation, coitus interruptus, and abstinence, which he called 'aktuelle', or current neuroses.

Freud began to believe that neuroses came from mal-development of a child's sexual growth. The trauma involved were internal within the stages of sexual development, oral, anal and genital. He asserted that these conflicts were present in all humans, but were exaggerated in neurotics. These became repressed perverse sexual impulses in the cases of masochism, sadism, homosexuality, exhibitionism, voyeurism and fetishism. He also emphasised the bi-sexuality of men and women as did Jung with his explanation of animus and anima.

THERAPEUTIC ANALYSIS
Freud conducted his own self-analysis, but later changed to agree with Jung that analysis should be conducted by another person, and that analysis was essential.

Tools used in analysis, methods to evoke communication of the repressed are:

SYMBOLS
There is a conflict between the meaning of Freud's symbols and those of Jung's. Jung regarded Freud's use of symbols as representations of what was known, especially in the area of sexual symbols. Freud took symbolism as a representation of something else in a more acceptable way to the ego. Jung, on the other hand, took symbols as representing the unknown trying to make itself understood. He considered Freud's use of symbols as signs. This seems to be a semantic argument which Jung used in order to claim his own special use of a word. Jung sometimes calls this the 'transcendent function', the power of constructive changes within the psyche.

DREAMS
Freud's interest in dreams started in 1892 and gave birth to 'The Interpretation of Dreams' in 1900. According to Freud, dreams are *'disguised, hallucinatory fulfilments of repressed wishes.'* These expressions of wish fulfilments dated from the person's childhood. Current trauma awake memories of trauma from childhood. They represent indirect expression of childhood wishes that had been repressed, and which would disturb the dreamer so much that he would wake up. Ideas are converted by the super-ego to acceptable visual images and symbolisation of sexual thoughts which would be distasteful to the ego. Those ideas are made into a coherent story, of which, the recalled part is the 'manifest content'. However, the disguised part is the 'latent content', the part that can only be understood with an analytical approach of 'free association'. Freud considered that the interpretation of dreams is *'the royal road to a knowledge of the unconscious activities of*

the mind'. Freud has to take credit for serious dream investigation, but his obsession with all things being sexual, misdirected his findings and conclusions, I feel.

Jung took Freud's views as a starting point for his own developments, adding the collective unconscious as a contributor to dream content, thereby adding far wider issues than sexual ones. His approach was more optimistic, believing that dreams are part of the homeostatic process leading to positive change. He believed that dreams are better utilised by using 'amplification' and 'active imagination'.

Amplification is allowing the ambience of the dream to embellish the whole experience. Symbols are taken as information from the collective unconscious and are explored as such. Active imagination is a state of relaxation, which seems similar to hypnosis.

ACTIVE IMAGINATION
Active imagination is described as a relaxed state where the patient is <u>almost</u> dreaming with his eyes open. It requires the active participation of the patient who is encouraged to become totally involved in a picture or any other stimulus which leads to an unconscious stream of thought, uninhibited by conscious directions. There is a great similarity to hypnosis in which the patient is allowed to 'free-associate' whilst relaxed.

The desired end result is the reconciliation of those unconscious thoughts with conscious realisation so that the conflicts which have caused problems are settled.

HYPNOSIS
In 1892, Freud abandoned the use of hypnosis, in favour of free-association , or so he thought! His definition of hypnosis appears to be the currently commonly misconstrued one of a power over people, depending on the patient's compliance and the perceived power of the hypnotist.

Hypnosis does not have to be formally induced; merely by lying on a couch, out of sight of the analyst (eyes closed), and being asked to recall, will induce a hypnotic state. It is highly unlikely that Freud stopped using hypnosis, but thought that he had. He used a different style which he failed to grasp, and in a more efficient way to encourage free-association. It is probable that the main reason for Freud's abandonment of hypnosis was more to do with the greater ease with which 'transference' is developed when the patient feels to be in the control of the therapist and therefore allows the feelings thus derived to be expressed more easily. By renouncing hypnosis, Freud probably reduced the efficiency of his analytical technique and hindered the development of the use of hypnosis in later years.

FREE-ASSOCIATION
Put simply, this is where his patients, out of their sight of Freud, would talk freely about anything that came into their heads.

TRANSFERENCE
This is assumed to be the emotional attitude of the patient towards the therapist. Freud's early model was that the relationship should be professional and objective rather than personal. Freud was allegedly detached but his own case notes suggest otherwise. He seemed to interpret information directly to his patients, and in doing so directly suggested causes to them, **arguing** until the patient agreed with his findings. This hardly represents an objective approach. However, he kept himself from public scrutiny by giving no personal details, having his letters destroyed, and so on. Perhaps this was to discourage other analysts from analysing him in the way he did to others such as Leonardo da Vinci and Hamlet. Perhaps he was aware that he was hiding a guilty secret that he did not want others to find.

SUMMARY
Freud's basic theory is that unpleasant experiences, fantasies, or impulses related to sexual activities or sexual impulses are repressed as a defence in order to protect the ego, and are thus made unconscious. However the repressed memory makes itself known to the conscious as unacceptable symptoms which relate to the original experience, but differ in their expression. His therapy aimed to bring

the repressed memories, and their associated emotions, to the conscious mind so that the subversive energy was disposed of. This process of gaining insight is abreaction.

TODAY

If you managed to wade through the very heavy stuff above, as a therapist you must be questioning the relevance of Freud and Jung's theories and how you can use them to help your clients. Ask yourself if the problems you treat all stem from childhood sexual conflicts. Question and question again what Freud's theories have done. Also remember my comments about repression and suppression being a translation error and possible meaning the same thing.

Please bear in mind that Freud lived from 1856 to 1939 and Jung from 1875 to 1961. Both men lived in different era and a different style of social life to what we have today.

Certainly a good point is that they started the concept of analytical therapy. However Freud's obsession with sexual conflict has led to the erroneous ideas about all problems stemming from sexual abuse.

Rather than being considered to be the mainstay of practice in dealing with problems, Freud, and to an extent Jung, should be seen as relevant to therapy as their surgical counterparts were to keyhole surgery today. They formed a part of the base of knowledge for therapy but reading the above will, hopefully, encourage the reader to critically consider some of the principles.

Can we assume 100% that Freud was right and should be followed as a force that is beyond inspection? My conclusion is 'no'.

Panic, Anxiety, Stress and Phobias

Although anxiety, stress, phobias and panic may be defined as separate conditions, the physiological and psychological responses that those conditions represent are very similar.

The fundamental drive of any animal, including humans, is the survival of the individual. Without survival there cannot be reproduction and therefore replication of the species. In order for a person to survive a life-threatening situation, he/she has to be able to run away from the threat, or fight it in order to gain an advantage, defend as a last resort or to stay still in the desire that the threat will not notice him/her and go away. This is the fight or flight OR defend or freeze response (hereafter just referred to as the flight or flight response). None of the above has to be a sole reaction, there are mixtures.

This arousal is brought about by the sympathetic nervous system (SNS), one of the two divisions of the autonomic nervous system (ANS). When a threat is perceived the SNS is activated. This results in various changes to the body's systems including:

- The release of red cells from the spleen in order to ensure that muscles needed for fighting or running are well provided with oxygen.
- In order to deliver that extra oxygen, the heart beats faster and blood pressure increases.
- Breathing becomes deeper to supply more oxygen from the lungs.
- Sugars are released from the liver to supply energy to the muscles.
- Blood platelets, which help the blood to clot in case of injury, are produced.
- Endorphins, natural painkillers, are produced by the brain.
- Sweating increases to help the body to control the extra heat produced by muscular activity.
- The digestion of food changes, sugar is metabolised faster to provide energy to the muscles, but longer-term digestion is slowed or stopped in order to release blood from the digestive system,

which can then be used to supply the muscles.
- Other 'long-term' processes are also suppressed, such as the immune system.
- Receptivity to external stimuli is increased.
- Blood flow changes from supplying the skin and digestive system, in order to provide muscles with a better flow. To help maximisation of that supply, the blood vessels in the skin and gut increase in size. As part of that process the blood vessels supplying the muscles become smaller so that blood loss is reduced in the case of injury, which is why blood pressure has to increase.

Although the above responses are triggered by neural impulses from the SNS, they are maintained by the endocrine system, whereby a series of glands release hormones into the bloodstream. The pituitary releases glucocorticoids, which convert fats to glucose and also suppress the immune system. It also releases adrenocorticotrophic hormone (ACTH), which stimulates the adrenal gland to release adrenaline which maintains muscular activity and an adequate blood supply.

In any organism the maintenance of this highly aroused state is unnecessary and expensive in terms of energy resources and bodily health. There is a counteracting system, the parasympathetic nervous system (PNS) which restores balance by, for example, reducing the heart rate and blood pressure, restoring digestion, stimulating tissue repair and storing sugars as body fats, and so on.

It is important to note that there are scales of reaction within the fight or flight response, which cover intensity and duration.

There is a need to differentiate between purposeful arousal and survival arousal. It could almost be argued that there can be conscious arousal, such as found in playing and with planned physical activity (e.g. sports), and unconscious arousal which is reactionary to a situation that is recognised or perceived as threatening, and which may be labelled as fear and/or anxiety. Therefore, emotional input, as an instant evaluation of the situation, is important. The fight or flight response can be brought about by the thought of a threat as well as an actual threat.

There are differences between a phobic fear, stress and anxiety which are important to understand. It is useful, in diagnostic terms to understand defined differences, but it is more difficult to accept that they have practical validity in terms of establishing treatment strategies. For example, one of the results of fear is a panic attack, and vice versa. Anybody who has witnessed, or experienced, a panic attack will know how much fear is involved. Agoraphobia will lead to a panic attack if the sufferer actually has to consider leaving the comfort of home. By definition, a phobia can be a fear of a panic attack.

Rather than trying to offer precise definitions for diagnostic reasons and semantics, I would rather consider the areas of stress, panic and phobias to be aspects of the same underlying condition, that of the effects of the fight-or-flight response within the variables of time, circumstance and intensity. This is possibly a somewhat controversial point of view which is in need of substantiation and justification.

If I take as an example a person who is frightened of flying, but has been pressured into taking a foreign holiday, in six months time, by her family. At the point that the holiday is booked it is likely that the person will feel panic. Building toward the holiday it is likely that she will feel stressed and anxious. This is because she has a flying phobia, and she will have to face the experience of flying, which she dreads. Assuming that she receives no treatment, it is highly likely that she will suffer panic attacks during the time between the booking and the flight. It is also highly likely that at the point of reaching the airport she will be prone to panic attacks.

All three symptoms will have been experienced, including degrees of both fear and anxiety. The cause, whatever it is, will have remained the same, with the symptoms being different expressions of the underlying problem. To label those symptoms as being different disorders seems to be improper for defining specific types of treatment. It would appear to be more accurate to label the disorders as differing modes of expression of the basic disorder. The example can be extended to cover a huge number of different situations such as crowds, spiders, needles and so on.

If we consider reaction to a stimulus, either real or imagined, over a time span, then stress becomes a state of readiness stretched over a long period, and is related to the unknown. A phobia is similar but is confined to an object or situation which can be defined. A panic attack is the heightened reaction to a stimulus, but where the reaction causes loss of control rather than an improved coping ability.

Cause and effect can be either via a logical, or a convoluted link, however, the link is always being highly emotionally charged. For treatment it is necessary to uncover that cause, to defuse it and to reframe the stimulus.

Inductions

If you really want to scare your clients, use a rapid induction! Please never do this. These inductions are for show. For the most part they use the tactics of shock. Remember a part of the fight-or-flight response is that of freezing. These inductions are used by stage hypnotists and involve things like tripping people backwards, pulling arms to the ground and so on. Read about them as part of your academic interest but <u>never</u> use that type of induction with clients.

You want compliance from your client in order for you to help. Would you trust a doctor who, before examining you, burst balloons behind your back; or a hairdresser who produced a large pair of blood-stained shears rather than a small pair of scissors?

I feel that 'hypnotisability' tests on your clients are more to prove to the therapist that they can hypnotise somebody than for the benefit of the client. The client has assumed that you, as the therapist, will know the tools of your trade. Hand levitation and 'magnetic hands' may be used as shortcuts after a few sessions but they will take the clients mind to a place that they have visited before, a place of relaxation and compliance. If shortcuts are used too soon the client will confuse therapy with trickery and will be less co-operative than they should be.

I start with getting the client to push back in a reclining chair. This is less threatening than a couch or a massage table. It is more comfortable than sitting upright. The only time I have the client sitting is when we are dealing with flying phobias. Unless the client is very rich and would only travel in First Class, or Business Class, they will be sitting up on an aircraft rather than lounging back in a sleeper.

Next the client should be asked to take slow abdominal breaths using the diaphragm rather than the chest. The eyes should be closed. Lots of suggestions should be given at this stage. This means loaded instructions for the association of breathing with relaxation, such as,

79

'as you breathe in you will feel calmness flowing into all parts of your body and as you breathe out you will feel all tension is taken away with your breath and blown away from you.' The use of words like 'as' makes your words create a beneficial conditional response from the client. Other words are 'when' and 'now you are...' What you are doing is relaxing the body and mind together. You can tell your client the obvious, 'you are in a safe and secure place where all you are doing is allowing yourself to relax.'

Please avoid talking like a robot. This might bore a client into sleep but that is never the desired outcome. Some therapists talk in a bizarre way using a monotone and droning on. Use your voice to communicate with the client in the same tone that we all heard our mothers and fathers use when they were telling us bedtime stories. Never loud, always soothing, but colourful. The word 'big' is said in a big way whereas the word 'tiny' is said in a soft, almost whispering, tone. You must use a rainbow in your speech rather than drawing pictures in monochrome. When asking a client to gently breathe, you take a softly audible breath at the same time and in pace with the client. Likewise when you ask for the release of the breath. It becomes like hearing wave lapping on a beach.

Then you can bring the imagination into play. The client relaxes somewhere. A beach or a spot in the countryside or in their garden. Some people worry about locations. I remember that I avoided beaches as a location completely after the tsunami in Indonesia because any beach reference would have been associated with horrific visual images gleaned from the media.

Bring the location to life by asking the client to imagine sights, sounds, smells and feelings. This captures most of the sense modalities and will thus apply to the vast majority of people you will see. I like to repeat this part using different things to imagine. For example 'imagine you can see the waves gently lapping on the shore' is followed, in the next round, by 'imagine you can see little yachts sailing out on the water' and so on for the other senses.

Next the process of Progressive Relaxation is introduced. Always start with the head and work down to the feet. Why? If you have a cat or a dog, stroke it from the tail to the head and it will become unsettled. When you stroke from the head to the tail it becomes relaxed. This happens even if you do it above the fur. The same thing happens to humans.

The reason, I am sure, is because when we were being suckled our mothers would stroke us from head to toe. The mothers of cats and dogs will lick down the body in the direction of fur growth. It is more relaxing for your client when you move in that direction verbally.

Part way through the Progressive Relaxation, affirm hypnosis. I say, after they have taken the breath into the stomach, ' as you breathe out you drift deeper and deeper into hypnosis...NOW'. This a) Confirms that they should think they are in hypnosis and b) that they will be deeper after the word, 'now'. It works because clients are never sure if they are in hypnosis. You, the therapist, are working against preconceptions and misconceptions. Now you continue with the rest of the Progressive Relaxation.

This is the induction completed as far as it is needed for analysis. The client will deepen automatically when they start to recall events. Memories will take them to places and emotions they have stayed away from.

For suggestion therapy it is a good idea to give suggestions and then do a deepening routine before repeating those suggestions with variations. This creates a sense of intensity and credibility with the client.

For analysis, you ask the client to recall after giving them the approval to say anything that comes into their head no matter if it seems insignificant, irrelevant, shocking or embarrassing. You would have explained, when outlining the procedure, that 'there is nothing I have not heard over the past x years.' Rather than a boast, this is part of developing their acquiescence.

81

Your job is to record everything that is said in your notes with symbols for emotional outcomes without reaction or response that the client can be aware of.

After the first session you can repeat the first induction in its entirety, shorten it to breathing and Progressive Relaxation or just allow the client to assume induction after reclining, breathing and moving the mind back. What you do is within your judgement after the first or second session.

There is no magic in the induction other than, metaphorically, guiding the client by the hand to a place where they can open up their memories and emotions.

When people ask me how long it takes to learn how to hypnotise somebody then I will tell them, 'two minutes; but it takes years to learn how to use it correctly to help somebody.'

PART FOUR

Problems and Treatments

Please note.

Obviously there are many problems that have been left out of the following list. What I aspired to do is describe a broad spectrum of problems that should point the therapist in a direction to follow. The diagnostics and treatments suggested are to be only carried out at the discretion of each therapist and no responsibility for suitability or effectiveness of recommended strategies can be assigned to the author.

Abuse

To base therapy on the principle that most, if not all, clients that you will see have been sexually abused is a dangerous foundation. The Freudian idea that abuse, usually sexual, is repressed is a strange one.

I have seen lots of clients, but I have yet to meet one who had been sexually abused and who did not consciously know it when they first walked through my office doorway. The one thing that they had in common is that they had not told very many people, if anybody, about it. Very often sexual abuse is a trauma remembered but rarely spoken about.

This is suppression rather than repression.

The topic of abuse opens a multi-dimensional area. There are different forms, different shades and different ages of abuse.

- The different forms include emotional, physical, sexual and a mixture of some or all of those.

- The differing shades are intentional and unintentional by the abuser.

- Differing ages have an impact on the outcome.

These factors give a complex mixture of effects and outcomes that must be understood by any therapist. To this end, each type of abuse is given a separate heading.

Abuse, Emotional

"A sneer is the weapon of the weak." James Russell Lowell (1819-1891) American poet, critic and editor.

(See also the heading titled Confidence.)

The purpose and motivation for the abuser is to diminish the self-respect of the victim. The abuser will rarely recognise what is being done and carries on regardless. The ultimate end can be the threat of, and the carrying out of physical abuse.

Typically, the abuser will tell his partner (although this is something done by both sexes) that she is ugly, lazy, selfish, sexually unattractive (although also allegedly unfaithful), lousy in bed, a poor carer, a bad cook, a useless person who is unintelligent and so on. What the abuser wants is for his partner to believe that the only man who will tolerate her is him. He will often tell the victim that she is lucky to have him because she would never find anybody else who loved her as much.

This gives the main clue to the abuse. The man is jealous and wants to control his partner. This reflects his own unconscious feelings of inadequacy.

The person who will see a therapist is the victim rather than the abuser. It is impossible to treat a third party, no matter how much it is needed. The resolution should be with the abuser rather than with the victim.

At some point the victim might bite the bullet and leave. Then the abuser might see a therapist to work some sort of magic to persuade his 'ex' that he is making efforts to 'change' in the hope that she will return.

Therapy is never able to change circumstances but it can change attitudes towards them. The role for the therapist in this scenario is to built confidence and self-esteem with the client. You should never offer advice about what the victim should do to the abuser. The obvious thing would be for her to leave but this goes beyond your brief. In building confidence the victim should be able to make up her own mind to do so.

In pretty much the same words as above, a child is given the impression that he/she is a disappointment. A child is told that 'standards' have been not met, whatever those standards are and by whom they have been set. Sometimes this is well meant as a spur for the child to succeed where a parent failed. Sometimes it is the sort of rough control that bad dog owners exert on dangerous breeds. This is never kind, only controlling.

Sometime sibling rivalry will have a bearing especially with an older and bigger sibling. There is a drive to eliminate siblings in order to gain better recognition and, in primeval terms, a better parental protection. (More about siblings later.)

Then there are, what can only be described as 'Queen Bee Mothers'. This is the phenomenon whereby a mother is unable to release her control of a daughter, even when the daughter has grown up. The mother wants to vet boyfriends and can become very insulting about her offspring. Getting a daughter to gain control is difficult because she gets stuck in the trap of 'having' to do things out of duty because that controlling person is the client's mother and 'good girls have to do what mother thinks is best.'

The therapist's route can only be to break the tie and this, perhaps is beyond the level of influence that a therapist should offer. If the only way to ensure that the client is liberated is to destroy a relationship and thereby upset the mother and by imposing a sense of guilt on the client, then you must think long and hard before taking on the victim as a client.

The following are quotes from the mother to the daughter as indicators that this problem is occurring:

- You shouldn't have done that.
- You are weak.
- Should have listened.
- You are collecting ammunition against me.

Within the problem there is a sense of the mother living vicariously through her daughter. She has to sanction every decision. Sometimes the mother's actions are a reflection of the mother's own mistakes.

Bullies obviously fit into this category as well as physical abuse. They pick on differences that they see. They could be racial differences, glasses, ginger hair, being too tall or too short, acne, a limp...you name it! If somebody is different in any way they can be excluded from the group. Albino blackbirds are pecked to death. It seems that humans who spot somebody who is seen as something other than the group is, treat victims in the same way.

One wonderful story to build confidence in bullied people is the Hans Christian Andersen story about the ugly duckling. Remind your clients that what was perceived as different and a social pariah was, in fact, a young beautiful swan who grew to be bigger, better and stronger. The ducklings grew to envy the hero. This is a powerful metaphor.

Then there is emotional abuse by authority figures:

Creditors
Unpaid creditors become impatient and often threatening in their attempts to recover money that is outstanding. Although physical abuse can occur, it is illegal so the verbal threat is used to intimidate.

Teachers
In places of education the teachers can be as intimidating as the peer group bullies of pupils/students. This can be seen as an admission of a loss of control by the teacher who has to use abusive tactics to feel better. You will never see these people as clients but you will often see their victims. It is interesting that many teachers have had bad

experiences at the hands of bullying teachers when they were younger. The positive motivation is that they want to be good teachers to demonstrate how it should have been done.

Emotional abuse will have changed a client's beliefs about themselves. The need is to help the client to change those inner beliefs and to set new ones by clearing out the emotional damage that has been done. The therapist should allow conditions where people can talk about the abuse and its effects when it happened and the current consequences in their lives.

The main part of therapy for the victims has to be building confidence, self-esteem and self belief so that they can stand up to the unwarranted criticism and to see why it was, and is, erroneous. Your job is to empower the client, to create a sense of pride in what the person is and in what he/she can achieve.

Abuse, Physical

Sometimes it is possible to see trauma marks on a client's face, neck or throat when they are in hypnosis. Speculating about the reason for this is difficult. Perhaps they have been caused by an emotional response indicating that something has happened but is held secret as happens sometimes with blushing. Maybe it is caused by blood flowing more freely to damaged capillaries in the skin when the client is in a heightened emotional state. It is even possible from time to time to see whether the bully was left or right handed by location of finger marks.

Domestic violence
Most often the therapist will see a client who **was** physically abused in the past rather than somebody who is being abused when they seek your help. This is because people who are being harmed are usually too frightened that the abuser will discover that the hurt is being made more 'public' and will be made to become even more violent. The client feels trapped in a situation that needs a radical step to find resolution.

The clients you see will probably be in a situation where the past trauma resurface because of contact with, mention of, or a reminder of the abuser, occurs. Even if they are in a safe relationship the echoes of the past can seem to be made loud through circumstances that recall the past, or perhaps there is a reminder in her new partnership. This might be the marriage of one of the children or the birth of a grandchild and the subsequent increased likelihood of meeting the abuser. It can even be when stress levels rise so that the client feels threatened even if there is no threat.

Mothers can be willing to put up with violence if her children are safe and if they have nowhere to run. They will be much more able to escape if the violence happens with her children.

Although I am writing about women being hurt, domestic violence can also involve men being hit and hurt by women. Men have a better chance to escape but that often involves leaving children with a violent person and the problem is left unresolved.

This is also an issue in gay relationships where partners can become jealous of ex-partners or of new friends.

Again the dilemma is in treating a victim rather than the perpetrator. You, the therapist, will be unable to treat the anger and many other issues of the instigator. You can only assist the victim and this involves you moving outside of your remit.

However, assuming that the victim is in a new situation and the problem involves coming to terms with new relationships, then we can help by putting the ghosts to rest and enabling the establishment of a new level of trust in the current partner.

Bullying
The word implies school children but it should be seen as a general term covering siblings, adults, authority figures and so on. A husband or wife can bully a partner. They can bully their children. The children can bully their siblings. Children can bully other children or older people.

The cliché says that that abuse is perpetuated by victims. Perhaps in bullying this is more apparent. A boy who is bullied by his father is unable to retaliate with him but he can take out his anger and resentment by bullying another boy, or girl, in the household or classroom.

As stated before, many times, you will only be able to help victims rather than perpetrators.

Self harming
Self harmers are at war with their bodies! They feel the need to hurt and damage something that has brought emotional harm. This self abuse can follow on from other abuses that the client has suffered and the task of the therapist is to bring about an emotional reconciliation

between the client and the client's body. Often, self harming can reflect sexual abuse.

You need to ask which areas are being hurt. They can include arms, legs and breasts in the main, sometimes genitals. These will indicate parts of the body that seem to have been 'guilty' in encouraging things to happen! It is about guilt. It is a way of getting the client's own back.

Suicide or attempted suicide can fit into this category as well. If you are unused to dealing with this type of client then you **must** refer him/her to somebody who can help. If you are negligent in your therapy and the person actually does commit suicide then you have a liability for what happened.

Abuse, Sexual

Although I firmly believe that sexual abuse is never the cause of every problem that you will encounter, you will meet many clients who have been sexually abused.

The spectrum is a broad one covering incest, rape, under-age sex and paedophilia.

If your approach to the client is one that creates trust and honesty, an abused client will volunteer the information very early on. Freudian views would state that the trauma has been repressed, forgotten consciously, and that analysis will uncover the hidden memory. My view is different. Such upsetting events are remembered but seldom talked about through embarrassment and shame. When given an unconditional and sympathetic listener, the client will let those memories out into the open. The client who tells you that they have no early memories is using a defence that they have honed over the years. The truth is that they have one major memory that dominates and to tell friends and relatives bits of truth surrounding a 'shameful' trauma might lead to the need to confess all.

Those people know that you have heard similar stories many times and that you will be able to release the demons that are held.

If there are such things as shades of abuse then it is possible to recognise that a ten year old boy showing his penis to his eight year old sister is more akin to childhood curiosity than incest, although the effects on the girl might be intense. If a client tells you that such a thing was the cause of a problem, then that person feels that they were abused.

A thirty five year old father asking his eight year old daughter to touch his penis is abuse, without any doubt.

Rape is bad enough, but then there is rape by a family member.

Sometimes there is the rape of a daughter by other men with the compliance and consent of her father. Sexual abuse covers so many different areas that are horrific to hear about but you must be able to seek the release of the victim from the mental and physical chaos that follows.

Guilt is a huge issue. The power base of an abuser is the creation of a feeling of collusion in the victim. This will include feelings of guilt at complying if it recurs when the child realises that it was something that should never have happened more than once. "You wanted me to do it and if you tell anybody then I will explain that you made me do it." This is a typical line from an abuser whether father, brother, grandfather uncle or neighbour.

One quote I heard from a victim was, "But I have to love him because he is my father!" This was when the father made his daughter feel so guilty and suicidal after years of abuse and when taken to court by the police, she refused to give evidence. He was jailed, however, for the abuse of other young girls.

It is necessary to know that young people are prey to abusers. As a species our genitals give pleasure from an early age rather than when we have wedding rings on our fingers! There can be an immense sense of guilt at the innocent feelings of pleasure felt by the victim given by the cynical and selfish activities of an abuser. "I feel sick because I let it happen. I must be evil because I let it happen so many times." Abusers know what to do to create a sense of safety for themselves and the price is always paid by the victim. A young victim is always innocent despite what has been suggested by the abuser.

The sense of guilt continues into adulthood. Victims can move through periods of extreme promiscuity as they look for the positive and powerful effects of control of a man in return for giving sexual favours. Doing this hurts the pride of the woman, however. The after effects are usually that the man will run a mile after the sex and the woman feels rejected and hurt. In order to build herself up again she offers a different man sex in return for the short-term compliments and charm, until he has had his pleasure and runs away.

The scenario continues. Sometimes this cycle of events is done in a haze of alcohol and another series of problems is created. The client needs to know that she is not alone in having this experience. It has happened to many women like her. I explain that nobody has a gauge like a mileage gauge implanted on their body. If she is in a serious relationship then her partner would never know how many men she had slept with. It is about your client being able to put the past into the past and to live her life in the present and future free of guilt.

Then there is the opposite effect of frigidity which shows as a refusal to have sex for the pleasure of another person and/or the victim. Her experiences as a child put her off the idea that sex is pleasurable; she only connects sex with feelings of guilt, shame and filth. Her man is frustrated so he will buy her gifts and flowers in the hope that she will give in. Of course this replicates the probable gift-giving of her abuser.

Sometimes the effect is vaginismus where the vagina tightens in order to prevent penetration.

Your client, by getting rid of those feelings of shame, can accept that her partner wants to share something special with her rather than **use** her body for his sole pleasure. There is something different about a relationship that is for the growth of two people in harmony. You can explain the difference between a symbiotic relationship and one that is parasitic.

A shark has a symbiotic relationship with a pilot fish. The shark's presence protects the pilot fish and in return the pilot fish consumes parasites that irritate the shark.

Yet, a parasite uses its host for its own benefit. A mosquito sucks the blood of its host and is never concerned that the donor might die from malaria. An abuser is a parasite. A loving partner will form a symbiotic relationship with the person he/she loves and respects.
Note: Never assume that abuse is the domain of males. I have treated

men and women who were abused, as children, by their mothers, aunts and babysitters.

The treatment is about changing outcomes. The client needs to release the shame and guilt. He/she needs to know that they were the victim of a sexual predator. The new outcome has to be that those parasites are a breed apart and that love and respect will come from a secure and loving relationship where sharing, rather than taking, is paramount.

Anger

"Must give us pause." Hamlet.

BEFORE TAKING ON A CLIENT WHO HAS AN ANGER PROBLEM, GET THEM TO PROMISE THAT THEY WILL AVOID HITTING YOU! AS SILLY AS THIS SOUNDS, THEY NEED TO COMMIT TO GETTING BETTER. SHAKE HANDS ON THE PROMISE BEFORE PROCEEDING.

The formula is simple; when people lose their tempers then they lose relationships, lose job, lose friends and lose advantage. Put briefly, they can lose everything that is precious.

Anger is often a displacement of feelings towards somebody who represents a person or people from an earlier trauma. We need to uncover who, in reality, the angry person had the issue with and then defuse the reaction to be more appropriate in the current situation.

The earlier perpetrators of the original situation will include bullies or dominant siblings. Perhaps it came from authority figures including parents, teachers and members of the clergy.

The process of displacement, or misdirection, that you will find could be when a client becomes angry with his/her partner. This might be venting feelings that he/she developed as a child towards a dominant or bullying parent but was too small to express them. When he/she grows into the position of having a partner who, for whatever reason, reminds him/her of their childhood, then that bottled up rage detonates and hurts the person he/she loves the most. This never justifies the anger but shows that it is often inappropriate and totally out of place. Nor does it suggest in any way that the man/woman should become angry with his or her parent(s).

As a mature person he/she needs to understand what happened in his/her childhood and come to terms with life as it is in the present day. All the client wants, like everybody else, is love and to be seen in a positive light. That can never come from expressing him/herself in an angry, violent or verbally abusive way.

Likewise, a person who becomes angry with their boss might object to being told what to do in a way that is critical or otherwise hurtful.

Nobody likes an angry person and you must be objective in dealing with them as clients. The wife beater, the child hitter and the bar fighter are never to be admired but your help will come to the rescue of their victims, indirectly, as much as it will in treating the client's problem.

We have to become used to living in a society that uses different laws to those of the fang and claw if we want to live in peace. Anger is potentially the most dangerous inheritance from our primeval past. Back then we had to protect ourselves from predators, including other humans. We had to hunt for, and kill, our prey. We had to use adrenaline to run faster, punch harder and frighten away those creatures we were too weak to defend ourselves against.

In our more recent history, the war cry, the threatening gestures in battle, and the intended intimidation of others, was vital to staying alive. How inappropriate those things have become in a bar, in an office or at home!

You should ask if alcohol plays a part in the angry person's life and if is does, it should be avoided or excluded and your therapy should look in the direction of finding why the angry clients needs to drink to excess as well.

When people drink and lose control there is a temptation to express those frustrations on the nearest person physically or emotionally. Just after Christmas is a busy time with clients who have wrecked lives by drinking too much and expressing otherwise suppressed feelings toward others. Sometimes people will look for a fight to impress their friends. Bar-room brawls will have bad outcomes because when inhibitions are blanked out by alcohol then there is nothing left to moderate behaviour that can lead to shootings or stabbings.

The objectives in therapy are to get your clients to:
Uncover the underlying cause of the anger. Rather than treating the outbursts with coping techniques, explore and re-explore the cause. Look at the client's early life from young childhood to late teens. Who bullied the client? How did the client respond? How does the person or the persons your client becomes angry with reflect those earlier experiences?

Answers to find:
Does your client judge people quickly?
Does your client carry grudges?
Can your client listen to what is said by others or do they jump to conclusions about what **might** be said?
Do they understand that out of control behaviour hurts the client as well as the victim in the long run?
Can they 'negotiate' an outcome that is acceptable to the parties involved without forcing opinions?
Would the client prefer a cuddle with their partner to an argument?
Can they walk away from a fight?

STRATEGIES FOR TREATING ANGER

After finding the real cause of the anger in the clients' pasts there is a need to place that cause into the past to enable a different approach to the present and future.

Chairing
Chairing is where the 'angry' person imagines the person at the heart of the problem to be sitting in a chair facing them. Then the angry clients express their feelings out loud at the imagined person.

They tell them what happened and what the outcome was. Then they explain how they have regained control and now that they know who was at the cause, they can stop showing anger at the representational victim or victims.

This works for a number of reasons:
- The clients nail the cause to the real perpetrator rather than the current victim.
- Then there is an acknowledgment that they have misdirected their anger to the wrong recipients.
- It also gives the clients the sense of a different outcome now that they have corrected the situation.

Throwing bread for ducks.
This is a physical release of pent up feelings. Screwing up a slice of bread into a ball takes effort, and throwing it away releases more physical effort in a strangely humorous way. Another benefit is that the client will have to walk to a pond, river or canal to do this. This takes more physical effort and gives cooling-off time, both of which should be beneficial.

Make comparisons.
You, the therapist, place two similar objects side by side on a low table. Get your client to imagine that one of them is a precious memento of somebody special in their life, perhaps a grandparent. The other is something that has no value.

Ask the client which object they would throw in the height of an angry outburst. They will choose the object with no value. Then you can point out that **even in a rage they have the ability to make a rational choice.**

This means that where they previously lost control, they actually possess it. Clients will take this notion away with them and should be able to control their feelings long enough to calm down when next challenged.

Gaining control for an angry person takes time. Ensure that the clients have reached a safe frame of mind before discharging them from therapy.

Anxiety

You will rarely treat anxiety as a problem but will hear the term used very often.

Anxiety is a broad definition that has to be broken down into more specific things. It is like the term 'music' that covers everything from Bach to Heavy Metal. If somebody tells you they like music you would ask them which type of music they like.

So, when a client tells you that they suffer from anxiety you need to elicit what the real issue is. Maybe panic attacks, perhaps stress, sometimes phobias.

The exception might be 'anxiety attacks' which is an alternative term for panic attacks, but during the Introductory Consultation you will clarify what is meant.

The client will use broad terms, you must take those terms into language that will be used for treatments.

Atavistic Phobias

Atavistic phobia is the descriptive word for phobias towards things that we seem to be predisposed to learn to dislike quickly. We seem to be able to very easily fear certain things that were dangerous in our primeval days on earth, and still are in certain places. They include spiders, snakes, lizards, frogs, birds, heights and water. The fears that our cave ancestors developed are still in the system.

It takes a scream from a mother to create a spider phobic. The fear caused by the scream is displaced onto the object that caused it. The same thing happens with snakes but the worry and concern of a parent, friend or sibling whilst walking through a field is strong enough. It could be a television program that dramatises a strike from a snake at the camera or a horror film in which snakes become man eaters.

A phobic reaction can be caused by having a frog dropped down a shirt or blouse. It is brought about by young fishermen throwing bait maggots into a person's face. It happens when non-swimming parents watch their children in a pool and keep warning them of the dangers.

Atavistic phobias are easily learnt, so the release from the phobia should be straightforward as well.

Your clients need to make friends with their enemies. Images that are held are so emotionally charged that it might seem difficult to contemplate making friends, yet is it easy. However, be careful in how far you take a client. You would never want a snake phobic to be so blasé that they would kiss a cobra. (I have been told by a doctor that many rattlesnake bites in America happen when men wish to kiss one to show how brave, or drunk, they are.) However, a snake phobic should be able to tolerate taking a walk in the countryside on a warm summer day without having panic attacks.

Sometimes the point at which the phobia started is remembered, such as stepping on a snake or when a brother dropped a spider down his sister's blouse. When the cause was at an early age then it is more difficult for the client to remember the actual cause. Coping techniques and a change of perception of danger are needed.

There must be a caveat about some spiders and snakes. Some are very dangerous. These live in hot places like Australia, America and South America and the Far East. To develop a tolerance without a sense of responsibility is wrong. Your job as a therapist will change if you have a phobic who is scared to travel in case they meet a very poisonous spider or snake. Now the job is to build acceptance within a framework of safety and caution. It is unlikely that your client will come into close contact with those dangerous creatures, but you must be aware of the possibility.

With the following, use analysis to discover the cause. This might be difficult with this type of phobia, but it is necessary. Then use visualisation and suggestions to resolve the phobia.

SPIDERS
Spiders look scary to phobics because they are fairly unattractive. They are ugly because they are a strange looking life-form with eight legs. However, they are more scared of the phobic! The person has the real decision about life and death and a book or a shoe quickly kills. Spiders want to stay alive and they will scuttle away to a safe haven. As they scurry they look strange because they have to navigate with those eight legs. In fact they are slow and jerky rather than fast.

The phobic needs to look at a spider in a different way; as a clown. They run around in a directionless way. They are similar to comedians acting out jokes when they run around a stage.

Their prey will be flies and mosquitoes, the real enemies to mankind. They are wonderful at looking after us because they prevent flies landing on food and infecting it with dog waste. They stop mosquitoes from sucking our blood which at best is painful and, at worst, gives us malaria.

Encourage your client to perceive a spider as some sort of guardian angel that sits on high. This is powerful if the client has children and worries about illness. The client can imagine the spider to have a smiling face as it would in a cartoon rather than the horror film face with venom dripping fangs.

You can tell your spider phobics my following true metaphorical story:

My grandparents were farmers in the early twentieth century. They were unable to afford pesticides, even if they had been available. They lived in an environment that was potentially dangerous. Cow dung, pig dung and chicken droppings were part of the scenery; everything that flies love to land on. My grandparents milked the cows everyday, and flies love milk.

The only protection available was the spider. They never caught any infections from the spiders and had a wonderful expression that would have dated back hundreds of years. "If you want to live and thrive, let a spider stay alive."

Spiders are our protectors against disease. The client may avoid picking them up and cuddling them, but because there is nothing to be afraid of, ordinarily, they can be picked up using a glass and a piece of cardboard to be released back into nature.

SNAKES
Fifty thousand years ago, snakes would have been a bigger threat than they are now. They would have been more numerous and medical aid would have been difficult to find. Adders are a protected species today. They have become fairly rare.

Snakes are either venomous or non venomous. In Europe, we have only one venomous snake and that is less of a threat than a cold or flu. Apparently, the last recorded fatality from an adder bite in the UK was over thirty years ago and that was a child.

Making friends with snakes is difficult because they are so difficult to find. With any snake, it is best to avoid attempts to catch or handle them. Most of the rare adder bites that have occurred followed when people have tried to catch them. They, like all creatures, will defend themselves when threatened. They have the fight or flight response as well as we do and, most often, choose flight.

It is a good idea to reassure your client that the risk that they will be bitten by a snake is tiny. Search on the Internet under Adder Bites, and you will see that their reputation as monsters is undeserved.

A good treatment is familiarisation. It is impossible and inadvisable for you to handle snakes in your office so encouraging them to visit zoos and looking at snakes will wear down the fear. If your client is able to handle a snake under the guidance of a keeper, so much the better.

HEIGHTS
Once again the warning has to be given that the aim of the therapist should be to enable a height phobic to cope when it is safe. This means that rather than getting a client to want to stand on the edge of a cliff, you should help that person to travel in lifts or on escalators.

Use analysis to investigate cause. This might be something that seems totally irrelevant to the problem so you will need to think fairly laterally as if solving a cryptic crossword clue.

Examples are being scared by a high slide in a children's playground, a fairground ride, being lost in a shopping mall lift and so on. It might be an over anxious parent warning a child, or adolescent about their concern at heights and emphasising the danger. Remember that atavistic phobias are easily learnt and the original incident(s) can seem trivial in hindsight.

What the fear has become is a phobia of being unsafe and feeling a loss of control. (There is more about Control under that heading.) The feeling might be an urge to jump from a height or that of falling off and crashing to the ground. It is unusual for a flying phobic to worry about heights, more about the loss of being able to control what is happening because somebody else is calling the shots.

A fear of heights can be dealt with by promoting a sense of control rather than the danger that would come with the loss of it. Thus a parachute jump is perceived as unsafe but a tandem jump is seen as safer. A bungee jump would terrify a height phobic unless they knew it was totally safe. That is why bungee jumps are well supervised and often take place after a peer has done one. Perhaps parachute and bungee jumps are beyond the desires of height phobics but they, as examples, show that a sense of control is vital for successful therapy.

WATER

You will see clients who want to be more confident with water. They might wish to learn to swim or go on boats. You need to know the limits. A non-swimmer should never feel so confident that they will want to go into heavy swells in the sea or jump into the deep end of a swimming pool.

Again you have to look for causes. They might be things like parental over-concern for safety, bad experiences in a pool such as being held under water by bullies, falling into lakes or rivers and so on. The trauma will often be connected to water and fear, of course, but there could be other causes.

They could be abuse in the changing rooms or being inappropriately touched by an instructor. It could be learning of a drowning by a child or adult, for example. Never assume a cause. The client must tell you in clear, or concealed ways that have to be clarified, what the root of the problem is.

The only way in which the client will experience a resolution is by getting into water. This should be the sole domain of a qualified and trustworthy instructor. You give the confidence and somebody else should give techniques and swimming expertise. If the problem started with abuse, the person chosen must be scrutinised. Never offer to take your client swimming yourself.

THUNDER AND LIGHTNING

I have seen older clients who were scared of thunder and lightning because they had lived through the Blitz during the Second World War. The flash of light followed by a bone shaking explosion is a description that fits bombing <u>and</u> thunder storms.

Playing fields also attract a sense of contagious panic, especially with parents watching children playing in wide open spaces at the beginning of a storm.

There have been beliefs that lightning will be attracted by mirrors, as if they can think, so the best thing to do is pull the curtains. If the client believes this, then that anxiety at having to rush around to close the curtains can heighten a fear.

Lightning is dangerous, for sure, but given the right actions to take during a storm we are all relatively safe. Deaths do occur but these usually involve people hiding under trees, people near water and people outside their homes, presumably watching the storm. Lightning is mostly a danger for golfers, cyclists, fishermen and campers, apparently.

An obvious thing to do before starting treatment is to study what to do to avoid being struck by lightning and inform your client. Being in a car is a good example. Then you can deal with the traumatic memories and defuse them. The aim is to enable your client to be safe and, at the same time, be able to tolerate the flashes of light and the claps of thunder. The War ended a long time ago but there have been terrorist and civil explosions since. If the client was affected by those and has projected the fear onto thunder storms this might be a sign of post traumatic stress disorder and should be treated as such. In other words the cause has to be identified and dealt with.

If it is to do with playing fields and open spaces then safety procedures must be adopted. Tolerance of the noise and light are something that is added to prime safety.

Bed Wetting (Enuresis)

When working with children a parent/guardian must ALWAYS be present.

If a client comes to you with a child who wets the bed, the first thing to do is ask if a medical professional has been consulted. Sometimes the loss of control of the bladder has a physiological cause and we, as therapists, are unable to offer appropriate treatment.

Assuming, therefore, that the cause can be treated, the first problem to overcome is a young child's lack of attention/concentration in a therapeutic situation!

The next thing is to discover what pressure has been applied to the child by the parents. Often bribes will have been offered, followed by threats on occassion. Sometimes children will have their beds fitted with an alarm that makes a noise if the child passes water! These would work if the alarm went off before the child wet the bed, but the alarm just screams out the problem to everybody in the household and can intimidate the child.

Nothing else has worked, so the therapist is approached as a last resort!

Make friends with the child. Show that you are human. The child is possibly embarrassed. You are yet another person who has been told the details of the problem.

Sessions should be conducted in a different time frame to that for other clients. If 15 minutes have sufficed for a session, never extend it to cover an hour. Formal inductions will rarely work but metaphors can communicate better with a young person. You want images of special helpers who wake the child BEFORE the bladder empties. You need to adopt the mind of a child in terms of what works. Remember the child's age. What works for a four year old will miss the mind of a seven year old.

What works well with a child who is known by his/her peer group to be unable to go on sleep-overs or to go camping is a method to show the peer group that the child has a knowledge that will enhance a previously damaged reputation. Parental inducements will only bring a child to level terms. His/her peer group will already have the train set, the fashion doll or the computer game. This information advantage can take many forms.

I have used 'magic' as a way out of this method. I am no magician but I have learnt three simple slight-of-hand tricks. You can find many on the Internet.

After making attempts with guards and helpers in the imagination of the child, then something different and special can seem to complete the therapy. Let me quote an example. A seven year old boy had never had a dry night. (The use of the word 'dry' is important because the problem is a wet bed. The positive aim is to create dry beds.) This young lad was proving difficult to help. One week I showed him a simple magic trick and he was impressed. He asked if I would show him how to do the trick so that he could impress his father and his friends. I told him that I would if he had dry nights. (I know that sounds conditional, but it was something he was desperate to learn, and he needed help.) He arrived the following week with a smile from ear to ear. He told me that he had been dry for four nights. At the right time he had woken and gone to the toilet. I showed him how to do the trick and I showed him a second trick. The following week, in order to learn the second trick, he boasted seven dry nights, and this was confirmed by his mother. I showed him how to do the second trick. The next week, after another dry week, was the last session apart from him telling me how impressed his father and friends had been.

My only question would be whether or not the first suggestions, in metaphor terms, about a guard waking him when needed had been brought to fulfilment by the inducement of the magic tricks or whether the incentive of the tricks worked on its own.

Blame

We seem to have a need to blame others for our own problems but sometimes those issues are of our own creation.

Yet you will rarely see a client whose problem is described as 'I blame others' but you will see clients whose issues have been derived from being blamed and who need to focus responsibility for their problem on a guilty party such as a parent.

We can use the process of blame in therapy, ironically. If a third party is to blame for a client's problem, then it can be acknowledged. However, the purpose is never to take that sense of blame to an extreme. It can be used as a bridge to release negative feelings BUT the person who is blamed has to be let of the hook in most cases. If a client's mother or father treated the client badly, then blame is appropriate.

What must happen, however, is an understanding of why the mother or father was like they were. Did he/she have a bad upbringing? Was his/her marriage bad? Did the client, as a child, add to the financial burden that was being carried? Was he/she treated badly by his/**her** mother or father? And so on. Was that person taking out his/her feelings on a defenceless victim as an escape from his/her own situation?

What you are exploring with the client is a reason and therefore an explanation. The harm will remain but in a diluted form. The important thing is that the client knows that what happened to him/her was the result of something beyond his/her control at the time. It was never because the client was intrinsically bad.

Blaming somebody in the short term is fine as long as the blamed person is let off the hook. In this way the client makes a 'firebreak' between their own experiences and their behaviour towards the next generation.

Assigning a cause of a problem to somebody and, at the same time, understanding why the person who caused of that problem acted in the way they did gives a context for the behaviour. In that way, the client is left feeling that they were innocent but that they became an outlet for the release of feelings held by the antagonist.

Rather than aiming to give forgiveness, the process offers understanding and most importantly a freedom from believing that they were a bad apple.

The exceptions are in traumatic sexual or physical abuse. We can blame the abuser but there is no need to let them off the hook because the chances are that the abuser will never be approached by the client ever again. To ask an abused person to understand the motives of the abuser is impossible and perhaps undesirable. The important thing is to stop the victim from turning the blame onto him/herself.

Blushing

There are some situations where our bodies seem to work against us as if they are run by alien forces. One of these is blushing. Blushing can be considered to be an unconscious expression of sexual attraction, guilt or embarrassment. It has been noted that when women talk to men that they find attractive, there is often a flush on the high chest. This is more obvious in women because they wear lower reaching tops. This can be seen as unconscious, yet overt, signalling.

Blushers can be helped in a number of ways. Analysis is necessary to find the original cause. Perhaps it started with being made a fool of at school, perhaps bullying or perhaps being put under pressure when older at work. Causes are difficult to find from the client so perseverance is necessary. Look at every point at which it might have started and also the points at which the reaction was heightened. Repetitions of blushing in different situations are like layers, and every time a blusher feels embarrassed, those times become a reinforcement of the problem.

With blushing, finding a cause is never enough. The client has to learn how to cope with a magnitude of different situations in their current lives.

Given that blushing can be regarded as a social signal it is necessary to change the response in the situations where the blusher reacts. The blusher feels anxiety at two things, the first being the situation and the second the blushing. Enabling the client to relax at will, helps. Teach them the breathing and posture techniques given later on and get them to practice.

Another thing to do is to ask them to blush. When the client *tries** to blush, it becomes an impossible task. This can help if the client is willing to *try** to make him/herself blush in those situations where they blushed before. There is nothing to lose. If they blush then nothing has changed. If they fail to blush then they have learnt a coping technique.

You can also enable your client to accept that they blush and that people have already noticed it. This means that there is little to worry about if they do blush. This, again, reduces pressure and reduced pressure equals reduced blushing. A positive feedback loop has been created.

The important thing is to get the blusher to perceive that blushing is a positive and pleasant thing. Women wear make-up to redden their faces and they do this on purpose to look more attractive. The cosmetics used are called blushers!

Why should a blusher worry? Encourage the client to stop worrying about blushing and to relax.

[* Please note that the word 'try' implies failure.]

Confidence

What a fool, quoth he, am I, thus to lie in a stinking dungeon, when I may as well walk at liberty! I have a key in my bosom, called Promise, that will, I am persuaded, open any lock in Doubting Castle. ~John Bunyan

I believe that 'confidence' is such an abstract thing that it impossible to give as if it were a substance. Loss of confidence, that of lack of self-esteem and a positive outlook comes from something that established those thoughts. So, rather than give confidence, it is better to remove the reasons why a person believes that he/she lacks confidence.

Very often abuse, in its general usage, leads to lack of confidence. The client's belief in him/herself would have been undermined in terms of appearance, ability or performance. You need to return the client to a realistic appraisal of those things by getting them to see that many things are said or done in spitefulness and thus, a negative self-belief is created.

The jealous person will talk about their partner being ugly or bad in bed. The bullying boss will insult even a brilliant performance because that boss wants to feel superior. That person is the one who lacks confidence and he/she wants to diminish the client rather than raise him/herself to a more noble height.

Get the client to put comments into perspective in order to realise that their confidence has been eroded by somebody or something other than him/herself. Collect the positive aspects of the client and frame them into a broad picture rather than a narrow one created by the person/people who stole their confidence.

This takes time and repetition. Often the client has lost confidence because negative things have been done or said over a long period of time. It takes a while to reverse those beliefs.

Create, with the client, positive affirmations about how good they are, how much ability they have and what they are able to achieve.

Be careful about complimenting a client of the opposite gender in case they inadvertently think that you have inappropriate desires. A person lacking confidence has rarely been complimented and is vulnerable. Confidence building has to be within the client. It is about their positive **self**-belief.

Highlight achievements. Sometimes the client will diminish achievements because they never recognised them as such. The people who have influenced them to think in a self- deprecating way would never have praised, only criticised.

Control

Control is a term within a broad spectrum. It is common to a lot of problems in that clients will fear a loss of control.

For example IBS sufferers will worry about a loss of control of the bowels when they are out. People who have panic attacks will feel out of control. Flying phobics are unable to delegate the temporary control of their lives to a highly trained pilot. A person in a poor relationship can worry about their inability to control what is happening and at the same time fear the dominant sense of control that a partner has taken. An overweight person feels ashamed at their inability to control their food input.

The list of examples could cover every heading in this list of problems of this book.

Control, or loss of it, is a major constituent of most of the problems you will be asked to treat. Giving a sense of control to a client is important to success in their situation. Treat each problem with that objective as a key goal to achieve.

Depression

Remember that there is nothing stable in human affairs; therefore avoid undue elation in prosperity, or undue depression in adversity.
Socrates

WARNING.
Before taking on a depressed client you need to know if they are receiving treatment elsewhere. Their doctor might have prescribed medicines or might have referred the person to a counsellor. Find out why they want to see you? Sometimes suicidal thoughts and depression can go hand-in-hand. Ensure that your client is somebody that you can help. If in doubt refer him/her to somebody who can. The stakes are high and you never have the right to experiment with a potentially suicidal client. Some people will see you as a last resort. Some people are depressed because they have a psychosis. Some will want a miracle. These people should be referred to a professional who is highly trained in these matters. Usually this means a referral from a medical practitioner who knows the client.

As a rider to the above, depressed people who are on medication will tell you what they are taking and what the dosage is. They will ask your advice about the medication and dosage. You **must** explain that you are neither a medical doctor nor a pharmacist, assuming that is the case, and that you are completely unable to comment. You might have views but unless you are suitably qualified you have no voice about prescribed drugs. Imagine your clients telling their doctors that their therapist gave advice about the doctors' abilities to prescribe!

It has been said that there are only two causes of misery; having things that we do not want and not having things that we do want.

The things that we have that we could live happily without are more than material things. To name a few, they include a lack of love, lack of confidence, lack of encouragement and the lack of recognition and support. Envy can also be included. This reflects a lack of self-esteem when we are envious of other people's success.

To name things that we want; they are money, happiness, fulfilment, success and peace of mind.

To be very trite, the best thing for a depressed person is a sense of well-being and cheeriness. When they wake up the day should seem a time to do things rather than to avoid another 24 hours of bleakness.

An analytical approach can uncover the causes and these can be dealt with and eliminated. A few examples of types are given below. These are far from being all-covering.

1. Clients who had no, or very little, encouragement from parents. If they achieved 95% in an exam they were treated as having failed because the expectation should have been 100%. This covers boyfriends/girlfriend, allegedly lacking beauty, wit or charm. So with so much criticism and the bar being set so high, it is little wonder that self-esteem seems like a dream rather than a reality. This type of client has to be able to look in a mirror and like what they see. The person needs to know that the sole judge in their life is them self.

2. Clients who are lonely. Remember that your job is to deal with the effects of this rather than act as a lonely-hearts agency. You can never introduce two lonely clients to each other in the hope that they will become buddies. You need to find out why somebody is lonely and then act to find a resolution. If the client is a widow or widower, do they need some form of bereavement counselling? If the answer is 'yes,' then refer them to a bereavement specialist.

3. If your client keeps failing in relationships then there is an answer as to why.

4. If family/work pressures are causing problems, then this is where you should look for giving assistance.

5. This applies to all the above as well. When a person sees their life as

too complicated or too troublesome to deal with then the blackness of depression can overtake them. There is always hope but it can take a lot for a person to see that as an option.

When the past is dealt with then the client is able to look to the future. This is the key to relieving the depression. When all a person can do is look back with gloomy colours then they need to be able to see a brighter future in front of them.

I will use stories to illustrate the dumping of negatives and the acquisition of positives. One follows.

Describe their past as a dark, gloomy wilderness. They will agree. Ask them to look for the flowers that grew there. There should be some, but sparsely spread. They can see their bad experiences as big, aggressive looking cacti ready to hurt if they got too close. Get them to imagine their woes as big metal balls that are shackled to their ankles.

Then let them find a key. Lets them unlock the shackles. Get them to kick those metal balls full of their problems away. Then they can run free. No longer are they held back by dark thoughts. No longer are they burdened by the emotional debris that others packed into their lives. No longer are they held back in a lonely existence. And so on to suit the circumstances.

Bringing the bright things from the past and leaving the bad things behind, they can then walk into the future unencumbered. Then they can meet old friends and friends they have yet to meet. Then they can see a landscape that is bright and cheerful, full of flowers and birds and butterflies. And, above all, they can see a smooth path that leads to a wonderful future full of life and vibrancy.

The most important thing is they will have acknowledged a future. This will enable them to start looking forward rather than being stained by the gloom of the past.

Envy

"Envy consists in seeing things never in themselves, but only in their relations. If you desire glory, you may envy Napoleon, but Napoleon envied Caesar, Caesar envied Alexander, and Alexander, I daresay, envied Hercules, who never existed." Bertrand Russell

Envy differs from jealousy, although the terms are sometimes confused. Envy is the negative feeling somebody has because another person has something that the envious person feels that they lack. This could be a car, money, a partner or an attitude. Clients can be envious of another person's social standing or of their air of confidence.

This has implications in self-esteem and the client needs to make better comparisons or to be able to live with the assets, perhaps unrecognised at first, that the client has.

Everybody is different and comparisons are easily made that are hurtful. A girl who is told by her best friend at school that she is ugly might be envious of her friend's looks, but later on in life the Hans Christian Anderson story of the Ugly Duckling could become relevant. Perhaps her friend was envious of her in the first place because she was in competition for the attention of a boy.

One man might be envious of a friend's sports car, but perhaps that friend is envious of the first man's children who are transported in the slower, but safer, estate car.

Envy becomes relative. A millionaire has lots of money by definition, but does the millionaire have a contented life? After all, some millionaires keep chasing more and more money rather than, perhaps, being able to sit back and enjoy a quality of life in emotional terms.

If you have a client who is envious then they need perspective. They need to recognise the value in what and who they are and can be rather than bemoan the fact that they fail to match another person's life or personality.

Fertility/IVF

Sheep that graze in lush fields are more likely to produce twins.

Perhaps your client wants just one baby rather than twins!

The first thing to ascertain is if your client can become pregnant. There are medical problems that need the help of drugs or surgery. These are beyond our help.

What we can do is help the potential mother or father to relax, to change the way in which they are going about conception.

If we look back to our primeval selves, it made sense to breed when times were good and to avoid becoming pregnant when times were unsafe. If food was likely to become scarce through crop failure, bad weather or the migration of our prey then we became at risk from starvation and our subsequent predation by the large animals on the plains.

It seems to follow that a woman could, and can, be prevented from becoming pregnant by using the unconscious resources of her body and mind. If, during the bad times, she conceived then the embryo, and then the baby would be at risk. She would be at risk herself. If she died then she would eliminate all chances of breeding in the future. Nature is cruel and it is kind. It stands to reason, intuitively rather than rationally, that becoming pregnant or remaining childless is related to the emotional and security circumstances of the prospective parents.

This also, perhaps, contributes to a lower sperm count for stressed men.

You should discover causes of stress in the lives of your clients. Perhaps instability of the relationship, perhaps problems with his/her work situation. If there are work problems this gives you a direction. Is

121

the client able to overcome their stress because it is self imposed? Teach relaxation techniques. If stress comes from external causes then it is more difficult to change the circumstances but you might change client reactions.

Your introductory consultation should highlight partnership issues. Does only one partner want to have a baby? Is pressure being applied by the couple's parents?

Check if there is an obsession with timings and egg cycles. The pressure to conceive can take away the pleasure of sex and cause stress. Encourage your clients to make love rather than make babies. Good sex is a stress buster; bad sex that is set to a calendar causes anxiety and anxiety is a good form of birth control.

Teach both prospective parents how to relax. You are a therapist and you should be very conversant with relaxation techniques. Read the section on breathing, posture and language and learn how to pass these methods on to your clients. Get rid of anxiety. The clients should relax before they make love. They can, perhaps, share a bath. The couple could gently massage each other. They should encourage arousal in each other.

Your clients should go for the orgasm. This is as natural as it should be. There are biological reasons why a female orgasm contributes to the movement of sperm to where it should be. Even if the woman climaxes later than her male partner, there are ways in which a woman can still achieve an orgasm after him. Get her partner to do some work!

As strange as this sounds to your client, so put it in delicate terms, get her to lay in bed after making love. Douching away the sperm quickly is never going to help.

The clients should put themselves in the mental state where they think of the baby as a child. This places their minds beyond the conception and pregnancy.

Tell your clients these stories:

Remember the women who became pregnant after adopting a child. Why? They relaxed.

Remember the girls who got pregnant from having a one night stand. Why? They were having fun, they were relaxed. The last thing they wanted was a baby.

Your clients must stop <u>trying</u> to have a baby, then they can have one!

IVF

The above applies to clients who are using IVF. You can never offer miracles. People undergoing IVF treatment need to be able to learn how to relax. This is to help to deal with the enormous emotional pressure that those previous attempts to conceive, and possibly disappointments with IVF treatment have caused. Problems and guilt can come from previous miscarriages.

Sometimes the potential mother will feel herself to be a complete failure and disappointment and let-down.

Explain to the client that relaxation helps at every stage from egg collection to birth. Keeping positive, yet without false hope, is important. Get the client to visualise success. She must see the baby after it has been born as a healthy child.

Realistic optimism is part of setting a mental frame that can help your client to succeed with IVF. She might be a member of a fertility group. Contrary to what might be thought, other members of that group conceiving creates pressure because she is aware of the statistics. For so many successes, in her mind, there are so many failures. For her every other pregnant woman reduces her chance of being a mother. So let her think that a success increases her chances as the process she is going through has be shown to work.

Flying Phobias

"When once you have tasted flight, you will forever walk the earth with your eyes turned skyward, for there you have been, and there you will always long to return." Leonardo Da Vinci

It amuses me to know that airlines will run "fear of flying" courses that explain how an aircraft gets into the air and how it flies. They give potential passengers all sorts of information that a science graduate would be proud to know. What they can miss is that the "fear" they aim to address is an emotional response. By way of praise, some airlines employ therapists to help fearful people to come to terms with the psychological disturbances they feel.

In my office I have hundreds of post cards from flying phobics who I have treated. I always ask for a postcard from the first place they fly to after treatment. I have them from the four corners of the world. Yet, from the many people I have treated I have yet to meet a flying phobic who was actually scared of flying! Somewhat ironically, flying phobias seem to have little to do with flying but rather an emotional upset that has been displaced onto the idea of flying and aircraft.

During your introductory consultation, the time when you are able to ask direct questions, find out as much as you can about the client's flying history and what the circumstances were before and after the flights. What you are looking for are the emotional connections that were made.

It is very unusual that flying phobias are created by bad flying experiences. Very often they appear to be the result of the projection of unfortunate experiences which are separate to flying, which become emotionally attached to aircraft, or the outcome of flying. In order to treat such phobias it is very necessary to find the original cause of the feelings of distress or panic, and subsequently change the negative feeling about flying to positive outcomes. The process involves exposing the emotions which were a part of the original cause and thereby nullifying them.

The following is an invented case study to make the point. Although it is fictional, the details have been based on real experiences.

A female client recalled, in hypnosis, the time that she had used all of her money to buy a ticket to join her Australian boyfriend. In the process she had argued with her parents, and had left on bad terms. She was nineteen at the time. Upon her arrival in Australia she discovered that her boyfriend lived with his parents on a remote farm, and the social and natural environments were very hostile to her. She was upset, the relationship ended, but she had no resources to buy her return ticket. Her parents refused to lend her the money because they had warned her about going. After moving to a small town and working in restaurants for months, she was able to buy her air ticket back home. The net result was that she felt unable to assign blame to herself, her boyfriend, her parents or the seeming recklessness of her actions. She blamed the object that had transported her to so much misery, the aircraft. Thereafter, aircraft became objects of anguish, and she carried the belief that if she flew, she would end up in a new disastrous situation, translated as her relationship crashing.

After treatment involving her comprehension of her erroneous condemnation of aircraft, and therefore accepting her personal responsibility for what had happened, she flew happily! During the Introductory Consultation she thought the problem was caused by a fear of death; her phobia seemed to be a survival strategy. However she was really avoiding the 'path' to disaster, which could have been a snake infested forest, an earthquake, a spider bite and so on. In logical terms she was unable to perceive that the 'path', the aircraft, was safe.

Without doubt, what my experiences in treating flying phobics have in common is the emotional turmoil within the clients which was connected to the thought of flying.

Not withstanding that, flying has been perceived as a dangerous activity, perhaps because at one point it was! Within my own memory base there are horror stories of air crashes. For example, I was due to fly to Spain on a school trip. A few months before we were due to go, an aircraft flew into the Pyrénées, killing a party of school children. This caused an incredible amount of media coverage. We went by train!

Similar memories are also held by the parents of the phobics seen. The essence of danger is ever present although flying is the safest form of transport. There was a time when it was almost obligatory to buy insurance at the airport before flying! The coverage of major crashes becomes ghoulish because if a plane does crash, a large number of people are killed. This sells newspapers and gives the television news-rooms something to talk about. The results of investigations are rarely published.

We seem unable to dissociate our fears from those disasters in the same way that we seem to be able to dissociate the carnage caused on the roads from a personal worry about what might happen when driving to work.

The treatment of flying phobics
Treatment proceeds in an analytical way using hypnosis to assist a more emotional state of mind, and to facilitate recall. After, usually two, sessions, a clear picture starts to emerge about influences that have had a bearing on the client's current anxieties.

Flying phobia treatment has a unique quality for me in that it seems more appropriate to discuss influences with the client, rather than waiting for the client's own insight. Emotional values of past experiences are usually fairly close to hand, and by discussion, the client can make the quantum leap from effect to cause, and the further jump to the erroneous fear of flying.

Having defused the original cause, the process then moves in a more cognitive direction, to change the thinking process from one of foreboding and fear to one of anticipating the pleasure of the trip.

Very few flying phobics have had a direct personal experience of aircraft crashes! In life we witness very few, if any, real crashes. We hear about them if a passenger airliner is involved, or in fictionalised form in films or on the television. Most of us have seen footage of fighter planes being shot down in wars.

However, there is a fear of crashing that seems to stem from the history of flying; a developing technology comes from a series of failures but every day successes are forgotten. The fear also comes from the occasional highly sensationalised news coverage of current crashes.

People worry about other people flying; "phone when you get there to let me know you are safe." This heightens anxiety in a subtle way. In the most ironic way, aircraft, being the safest form of travel, have safety announcements before take-off! They are big and defy logic as to how so much metal can float in the sky, hence the airlines' courses. As an attachment object for other anxieties, they are perfect!

Flying phobics therefore make up the threat from their own imaginations, they imagine what might happen. This of course makes them ideal for hypnotic intervention. There is a passive level of fear that can be made active by the association of the imagined disaster of an air crash and the effects of early emotional trauma which have to be placed in a similar, but not identical receptacle. Flying phobics avoid flying where possible. Therefore if inner anxiety can be connected to an object that can be avoided, then it can be controlled.

Causes of flying phobias
There seem to be three primary causes of flying phobias which may be grouped under the main heading of 'control'.

1. "if only".
This is assigning blame to aircraft for bringing about a series of circumstances that were life changing. For example, "if only father had not flown to xyz, then he would not have met 'Jane', and my parents would have been happily married, etc., etc." "If only the honeymoon

had been better." "If only my husband had not travelled for his career."

"If only we had not moved (flown) abroad, then my husband might have drunk less, our son might not have been so treasured by my husband, etc., etc." Flying becomes a means to a less than desirable end. So, rather than blaming the father or husband, the aircraft took the responsibility for disaster.

Similarity of object/experience.

These are unconscious associations between fear and an object that is almost incidental to an event. For example, a child being trapped on a garage roof whilst an Air Show was taking place.

Culpability.

This is a fear from the risk of making, or potentially making, bad things happen to those people who are loved. Flying represents potential pleasure, so the phobic, in this case usually a mother, suffers guilt at the thought that she is endangering her loved ones because she is thinking of her own pleasure.

Control

The linking theme with flying phobics is that of control. With "if only", the inability to control external events is considered to be responsible for 'blame'.

Likewise with "similarity of object/experience". If a person trapped on a garage roof had been able to control the situation by getting down, there would have been no problem.

"Culpability" also shows the sufferer's inability to control a situation. Sometimes six-year-old girls assume that their father left home because they were not good enough rather than recognising the strife between husband and wife. If a little girl had been able to control her parent's marriage then the split might not have happened when daddy flies off to his new love.

There are consequences from having been controlled and the clients' desire to have control over themselves by avoiding feeling controlled by being in an inescapable situation.

Making new associations.
This is done by using hypnosis to take the client on their planned flight, from leaving home, travelling to the airport, checking-in, going through security and so on until they are seated on the aircraft. As part of the early part of the session, when they are relaxed, comfortable and feeling in control, they are taught the anchoring technique of touching an ear so that if they do feel anxious at any point during the flight, they can immediately regain control and feel relaxed.

They are taken through the sounds and sensations of the doors closing, engines starting, the plane pushing back and taxi-ing out. Suggestions are added about noises and smells so that they become more and more involved with what is taking place.

At the end of the runway a series of analogies is introduced, "imagine when the plane starts to accelerate, that you are sitting in a fast sports car. Nice feeling isn't it?" When the plane lifts off the sensation in the stomach is likened to the childhood pleasure of going over a humpback bridge in their father's car. Various explanations are given, such as the turns, quietening of the engine noise, the noise when the wheels are retracted and the flaps slide in. All of this is done in an experiential way rather than as a mechanical explanation.

Very importantly, great enthusiasm is injected into the tone of voice as the aircraft is described as being like a swan waddling across the top of a river until it takes off; then the grace of flight is added, that the plane, like the swan, has been designed to fly, that it is in its natural element. The word 'freedom' is also emphasised. As previously mentioned, control is a big part of the reason behind flying phobias, and to emphasise the opposite of control, freedom, has a very positive effect.

Dialogue then continues through the flight and the client is encouraged by suggesting a positive, proud and supportive look on their partner's face. They are taken through turbulence, comparing it to the bumps that are felt in a car on an ordinary road. The example of a drink in front of them is given. In turbulence the glass might slide by but it remains upright. The client is asked to guess how long a glass would stay upright in a car, even on a motorway. Suggestions are made about the opportunity to sit back and relax, perhaps watch a film, have some food.

Next the landing is portrayed, describing noises and sensations, and the arrival at the airport building. One of the most important parts is also one of the selfish parts! The client is asked to imagine that they are writing a post-card to me from their destination, telling me how much they enjoyed the flight. In order to imagine doing this, they have to know and believe that they really did enjoy the flight. The useful aspect for me is that there is non-intrusive feedback that they did actually travel, that they did enjoy the flight and another post-card arrives to put on my 'flying phobic' board.

In their imaginations the clients spend their holiday in a happy frame of mind, and then are flown back. It is important that they enjoy the return journey; I need to avoid the client lying on a beach happy with the outward journey but fearing the return flight.

Guilt

Who sets the rules so that when we break them, we feel guilty?

There are some things for which we should feel guilty and others where we have been told we should feel guilty because it makes others appear to be higher authorities.

This statement needs explanation. Murder, rape, abuse, theft and injuring others are things for which we are made to be wary of being found guilty by society in order to inhibit the crimes. However, we all know that people transgress.

However, when abuse victims are made to feel guilty in order to silence them to protect the abuser we can see that the guilt is misplaced.

When a victim feels so much shame and guilt with their bodies because they are overweight, or because their bodies encouraged abuse, that they take a knife and cut themselves, who is the real villain?

Likewise, to a lesser extent, people are made to give food emotional values of good and bad so that when your client feels guilty because she ate a doughnut, then something is wrong.

The affects are the same. The transgressor feels the same anguish as somebody who commits a crime in being caught. People hide chocolate as if it were an illegal drug.

Moderation is a better goal than mental turmoil with some things that are made to seem like a crime. Your clients might feel guilty that they released emotion with tears. What is wrong with that? Only the stoic nature of modern life is.

The ironic thing about therapy is that you will rarely, if ever, see the instigators of problems. They hide their guilt; some even languish in the knowledge that they have committed an offence and gotten away with it. They will never risk telling you, a therapist, what they have done that is really a felony.

Our task is to treat the effects on people and to work with the client by releasing guilt because the assumed guilt never existed in the first place.

Guilt and blame (see separate heading for Blame) have things in common. If clients feel guilty then somebody has blamed them for something. Perhaps the self-blamer is the client. If they have something buried in their past that causes feelings of remorse then they need to release the reason why.

A mother who miscarries holds guilt at being unable to bring a child to full-term. It rarely has anything to do with any factors other than nature.

A person who was driving at the time of an injurious or fatal accident will assume full responsibility. If there is none, i.e. the car was hit by a drunk driver then the driver needs to release the pent-up feelings of accountability.

If, on the other hand, they were the drunk driver then you might find the task less acceptable to you. Then you make a choice in the same way that a defence lawyer has to when defending a person that is thought to be guilty on the evidence.

IBS

Patient: "It's been four years. I get cramps and diarrhoea and it's just destroying my life."
Doctor: "Oh, so you just have IBS."
Patient: "Yeah, whatever. That's what doctors say when they don't really know what the hell is wrong with me. I don't want to hear 'just IBS' anymore. I want some answers!" Anon.

PLEASE NOTE. NEVER UNDERTAKE THERAPY FOR IBS WITHOUT CHECKING THAT THE CLIENT HAS SEEN A DOCTOR ABOUT THE PROBLEM FIRST TO ENSURE THERE ARE NO PHYSIOLOGICAL PROBLEMS..

In our primeval past, as weak humans, it made sense to hunt and gather in groups. If we were attacked by a predator then the weakest and slowest would be caught and consumed much in the way that we see on wildlife documentaries with wildebeests and lions.

We can loose weight by emptying our bowels, bladders and stomachs so it should come as no surprise that we can do this when frightened. As a part of the flight-or-flight response, when we are scared, stressed or panicky our guts still react in the same way. We divert blood from our guts to our muscles for running or fighting. We have no need to be digesting in a situation where if we are caught then we become prey to be digested by another creature.

Those situations can be replicated by the mind in modern times when going out of the house. Anxiety levels lift because the client is fearful to be away from a toilet; almost a self-fulfilling prophesy. It can be when in a cinema, theatre or on public transport when the clients feel that they would draw attention to themselves by either getting up to go to the toilet or by fouling themselves in public.

Again, analysis will help to uncover root causes such as being 'caught short' in a school assembly or when having diarrhoea as the result of a bug. If this happened on something like a honeymoon or camping trip, then never be surprised. The ironic thing is that IBS sufferers rarely embarrass themselves afterwards because they are well prepared with pills or they only go to locations where they know that the toilets are in easy reach. You should ask if they have ever, or on occasion, been in a position where the occurrence of being caught-short has happened. You might be surprised by the lack of answers.

The client needs to be able to handle the stress and the fear of the fear in public. After finding the cause and setting into the past, your job is to teach relaxation and coping techniques.

It is interesting when considering breathing methods that in diaphragmatic breathing, the diaphragm massages the gut from the top. The abdomen is pushed out by the muscle rather than by air in the lungs. This upward and downward movement eases food through the gut in the process of digestion in co-operation with peristalsis, the wave-like contractions of smooth muscles in the intestines. The relaxation also improves blood flow to the gut and digestion is more efficient.

There is more about breathing and relaxation techniques later.

Metaphors can help. The desired movement of the intestine can be described as the gentle flowing of a stream that was hitherto hampered by rocks and tree trunks. The story can tell of a smooth passage to the sea. This must relate to the symptoms described so that a match is made.

Analogies for the parts of the gut should help the client to identify with the story. Lock gates, crashing boulders, tree jams and so on will empathise when used correctly.

Insomnia

"There is a new cure for insomnia. All you need is a good night's sleep." Tony Blackburn

Rather than thinking about insomnia as a problem that involves failing to sleep or waking up during the night, think of it as a phobia. Our minds want to keep us safe and as a result, we can live on that switch of anxiety, or a heightened state of awareness of 'dangers' in our lives.

The bedroom, for an insomniac, has become a place where the client needs to live on a hair-trigger; where we become transported back in time to our primeval caves.

Find out what the pattern is. For example, does the client fall asleep and then wake up at the same time during the night?

Does the client fail to fall asleep?

Find out if the person sleeps badly in every bed, some beds or just one bed.

Then you can investigate why the person sleeps badly.

A question to which you should look for an answer is, 'what is the insomniac frightened of when they go to bed?'

It could be that it is related to neighbourhood noise or to young children.

It could be that the client is stressed and worried by the work or domestic situation.

It could be from a person hearing their parents arguing when they were going through a divorce.

It could be a sibling sharing a bedroom and wanting to live a different time-scale lifestyle.

Ironically, poor sleeping patterns can, on their own, be the cause of the anxiety that keeps people awake.

In short, keep an open mind. Never assume to know an answer without gaining all the information.

Address language of intent. Insomniacs will feel uncomfortable when going to bed. I have met some who would wake up, worry, go downstairs and sleep soundly on the settee. Is this really an insomniac or a bedroom phobic?

The need is to change the attitude of concern for the bedroom to that of expectation of a good night's sleep. That is done by making fundamental changes to the client's emotional view of the bed.

Your task is to break a cycle, or to stop a negative feedback loop. When the client has had a good night of sleep then they have a different expectation the next time they want to sleep.

I ask clients to make friends with their beds. They should go into the bedroom and talk out loud to the bed. They should tell it that is a place where they have slept well in the past, where they made love, where they made children, where those children snuggled into on Sunday mornings in the past and so on.

It is better that the clients do this when they are alone to avoid alarming other members of the household. Then they can start to perceive the bed and bedroom as a place of peace, security and good sleep.

You are helping your client to stop thinking that they will sleep badly by showing them that by changing their inner dialogue and their attitude to sleep, their problem is erased.

Things for insomniacs to do:

- Make appointment with thoughts for the shower the next morning. This puts the worry into the future so a calm feeling can take the moment.
- Keep a note pad by the side of the bed and write in the dark. If the problem involves remembering things to do, a note pad takes away the anguish.
- Eat a lettuce sandwich. Lettuce contains Lactucin, a natural sedative.
- Have a milk drink. Milk contains tryptophan, a sleep-inducing amino acid.
- Do the Explosive Relaxation exercise before going to sleep. (This is described later.)

Jealousy

"O, beware, my lord, of jealousy;
It is the green-eyed monster which doth mock
The meat it feeds on; that cuckold lives in bliss
Who, certain of his fate, loves not his wronger;
But, O, what damned minutes tells he o'er
Who dotes, yet doubts, suspects, yet strongly loves!"

Iago from Othello by William Shakespeare

Unlike envy, a jealous person is worried that something they love, whether physical, personal or monetary, will be taken away by somebody who is perceived to be better. A jealous person might be envious of another but the jealousy is directed at what is considered to be the possession of the jealous person.

Usually a therapist will see people who are jealous in a relationship. This signifies a lack of trust. Trust is the foundation stone of love. This is trusting that the partner will be faithful and includes a sense of security about the future. It also signifies a lack of confidence.

In primeval terms, jealousy would have protected the nurture of children. A man who left his mate for another woman would have left hungry children behind so the mother would have been wary of competition.

A woman who left her partner for another man would have left her mate and would have taken his children with her so the man would have been worried by attention to his mate by another man.

Jealous people want to fight. This is seen with young people who are taking early steps in mating routines when they are dating. They assume that competition has to physically fought off. It is also seen in the control of a partner by force as if training a wild dog to walk to heel.

A question to ask jealous clients is if they have been unfaithful themselves. Sometimes a jealous person will project their own behaviour onto a partner. If he/she has been unfaithful then it stands to reason, in their thinking, that their partner will do the same thing. Quite often the jealous person is the one that needs help to settle the relationship down.

Ex-partners can be jealous of new partners. This is when the 'ex' is considered to be a possession and that somebody else has stolen it. This applies to an inanimate object but never to a person. If a man or woman leaves then it was for a reason.

A difficulty for the therapist is when a client describes their partner's behaviour in the context of their own jealousy and it becomes fairly clear that the partner is cheating. What advice can you give? How can you avoid being judgemental? You <u>must</u> keep your opinions to yourself. Allow the client to reach his/her own conclusions. They may be no more right than your own.

There are clients who have a predisposition to jealousy from experiences in childhood, sibling rivalry and so on. Perhaps they had bad teachers who showed favouritism. You may have clients who have been cheated on before and who have developed mistrust as a protection mechanism.

You need, always, to look for root causes. You need to unravel the tangled knot in all cases before progress can be made.

You must build trust and confidence. This goes with self esteem. If your clients think they are inferior to a partner, colleague or a friend then they have to see why that thinking is false and destructive. Again relativity counts. The client will have attributes that makes them equal at worst to a perceived rival. With the client, find what they are and build self belief.

Memory

There are some easily taught systems that can overcome the problem of poor memory. Memory is built, as you know as a therapist, on associations. The one that I like is also based on associations, as are most of them. The following system can be taught to clients.

The base of the system is a set of fixed images that rhyme with numbers as follows:

> 1 bun
> 2 shoe
> 3 tree
> 4 door
> 5 knife
> 6 sticks
> 7 heaven
> 8 plate
> 9 wine
> 10 pen

Make the images strong. For me they are:

1 bun. A big Chelsea bun with currants and sugar.

2 shoe. A brown shoe with laces.

3 tree. The sort of tree that a child would draw. A big round green area above a straight brown trunk.

4 door. This is a green door in a frame that is set in the country. No house, just a door frame on its own.

5 knife. A big black handled knife that I use for cooking.

6 sticks. Like a wigwam of twigs as used in a Boy Scout camp fire.

7 heaven. For me this is what the clouds look like when you look at them from an aircraft.

8 plate. A round, plain dinner plate.

9 wine. A standard bottle with a blank label.

10 pen. A big fat fountain pen.

Method
Write a list of ten objects. This could be a shopping list or ten friends or ten random words from a dictionary.

Make pictures of the objects that link the number word, e.g. 1 equals bun, to the word you wish to remember, for example, worm. This might means visualising a worm eating its way through your bun. Make the pictures vivid in the mind.

Then do the same with the next number and the word that needs to be remembered. For example see a carrot poking out of the top of your shoe. And so on for the whole list. You will love this system!

Usage
This is useful for personal use when making a shopping list. It may be used for remembering key points if you or a client has to make a speech. The uses are many. The great thing is once learnt the numbers and their fixed images will always be remembered.

Mind Altering Drugs

"The best mind-altering drug is truth" Lily Tomlin

Clients with dependency on mind altering drugs are difficult to deal with. They live in a fantasy world where they partly expect you to perform a miracle and, at the same time, want you to fail so that they can continue but with the added bonus that they can state that even a therapist was unable to help. This buys time.

Alcohol, cocaine, heroin etc. are ways to escape from an undesirable reality into a, perceived, better way of life.

In order to help you need to uncover what it is that the client is escaping from. Perhaps it might be bad experiences in childhood; perhaps it is a need to escape from a peer group that set standards of drug/alcohol abuse as an entry fee.

The aim should be to get the client to see that the perceived 'better place' is a dark and miserable place and that life is better enjoyed in a clear-headed and sober way.

As with anger, drugs and alcohol destroy lives and relationships. Jail can beckon for theft or violence when the usual social norms are excluded. With younger people fired with alcohol and testosterone, the bestial drive to dominate and fight becomes paramount. This is seen with drugs such as cocaine as well as alcohol. Cocaine use leads to paranoia and this in turn, can lead to aggression.

The reason that clients dependent on mind-altering drugs are difficult is that they have usually been told to seek help rather than, as with most clients that you will see, be with you on a voluntary basis. Another concern is that your treatment will cost money and a dependent person, unless somebody else is paying, will find it hard to pass a shop selling alcohol or a dealer selling a fix in order to pay you.

Talk to your clients in positive terms. Congratulate them on progress and <u>never</u> criticise if they seem to slip off track. They will have been dry/clean for a period of time. Praise them. If they took a drink or drug then praise them for the time they were dry or clean rather than become the authority figure in their life who admonishes. These people need all the help that they can get. The help they are offered by local and government authorities seems to be rigid and lacking, in my opinion.

You might be the last resort and as such, the only hope. Of course there are some places that offer great help to get people off drink and drugs. You should aim to be as good as the best, if not better.

Remember that your client's life might depend on you. If you feel that you are unable to help adequately, refer the client to somebody who can.

Take the client through analysis to find what they are escaping from. This can be frustrating if the client is lacking a drive to be co-operative, but persist. When using hypnosis be careful that the client stays awake! The only two clients I have seen who fell asleep had so much alcohol in them, and alcoholics carry it well, that they could have fallen asleep on the main runway at Heathrow Airport with Concorde taking off above them. I always make it a condition that clients with drink or drug problems are sober or clean for each session.

Needles

Find out everything that the client remembers about their experiences with needles. Most of the information should be gathered before analysis takes place. Analysis is aimed at the release of the emotion connected to those bad experiences.

The causes will be one or more of the following:

Pain.
We are very able at focussing our minds and nervous systems onto a very small point. This lets us know if a mosquito is sucking our blood, but this is usually after it has. The feeling that we have can be pleasurable as in being gently touched and unbearable as in being stung by a wasp.

A needle phobic will put complete attention onto that area of skin where they anticipate the needle will enter. Our aim is to enable the needle phobic to dissociate. This can be done by taking the mind away on a task such as searching for a treasure chest on the bottom of a reef encircled bay. It can be done by getting them to imagine having lunch in an old fashioned Parisian cafe. Paris is wonderful for getting strong imaginative images in most senses. The accordion, the smells, sights of the Eiffel Tower, the tastes of food and so on. As a quick story, I once attended a Caesarean birth with a needle phobic who was also diabetic. She needed a needle inserted into her spine deeper than an epidural. Ordinarily she would punch any doctor or nurse who came within five feet holding a needle. In the operating theatre I took her mind for lunch in Paris. She was absolutely fine. After the baby was born an attending mid-wife told me off, in serious tones, because she had not been invited for lunch!

Being held down.
Some clients will recall being held down and injected. This would have happened in childhood where the inconvenience to a nurse or doctor would have made them impatient. The only solution, in their minds,

would have been to forcibly inject the patient, your client, in spite of the objections. The treatment needs to gain the client's acknowledgement that they are now adult and that medical staff will have more respect. This comes after defusing the original event. Strangely, needle phobics will often be fine with a dentist because they differentiate treatments. Dental phobics, on the other hand are usually good with nurses. This gives clues to cause and effect. Heavy hands by professionals will point a phobic in a direction.

The fear of something penetrating the skin and putting, perceived, 'nasty' things into the body. (Fans of Freud should read on!)
These clients will think that something 'alien' is being forced into their bodies. Perhaps badly informed about how an inoculation works, they fear disease, albeit by dead cells. The fact that the purpose is to boost the immune system is given second place in their minds. An emotional shift is needed so that serums are seen as stimulants to better health and wellbeing.

The bad press given to childhood inoculations and possible negative effects would also give mothers a sense of anxiety that is passed on to their children.

Witnessing 'bad' things happening.
Children and adults who witness other people fainting after an injection can develop a fear of something similar happening to them. The days of mass inoculations have probably passed but they can still happen in the Armed forces and in some schools.

The treatments for needle phobics should take away the sense of fear by building a positive outcome. This can be better health and teeth, the chance to travel to exotic locations. Injections, thanks to advanced technology in needle production and the removal of using needles more than once, have become pain free to a huge extent. One of the most annoying things to hear is when a nurse or doctor says, 'Just a sharp scratch.' To me, the words 'sharp' and 'scratch' suggest pain and hurt. Why do they do it? Maybe, 'you might feel a tickle' might be better.

Panic

Panic attacks are an uncontrolled fight-or-flight reaction, hence the word 'panic'. Sufferers will might feel faint, will have symptoms of a heart attack, dizziness, feelings of choking, and breathing problems; or a mixture of those feelings.

In contrast to stress and phobias, panic attacks happen at a point in time, rather than being continuous. Panic attacks can happen to people who suffer from stress and phobias. They can happen as a response to a known stimulus, or to an unknown stimulus when they can then be described as being 'out-of-the-blue'.

The feeling of panic is a cognitive process. The sufferer knows how they feel, and as a result fear the next attack. This fear of the next attack adds to the feeling of dread within the person's experience of stress, or strengthens the element of threat felt in a phobia. Being highly exhilarated during a bungee jump does not lead to a panic attack, but the anticipated fear could lead to one. However the reaction afterwards is one of intense excitement rather than panic, despite the physiological responses being identical.

There is a cause for panic attacks. Analysis should find that cause but it might, once again be very cryptic. The introductory consultation will give some clues but ensure that a full history is taken down. Clients will often be hesitant about talking about early experiences of panic at first. You have to get back to the real cause.

Once you have discovered what it is together with the client, then you can start the process of putting those experiences back into the past. The use of language, breathing and body posture (see later on) are paramount in treating panic. Clients can sustain their problems so unless you correct the structures of thought, breathing and posture that the client has, you will be swimming upstream to achieve a long lasting resolution.

Parents and Step Parents

This deals with the negative effects that can occur. It has no implication that all parents and step parents will create damaging behaviours.

Parental divorce in childhood.
Sometimes clients will consider themselves to be at the centre of blame for a parental split. 'If only I had been a better son/daughter, then daddy would not have left.' Although the logical part of the mind tells the client that this is seldom the case, the emotional component remains. The client needs to interpret the mistaken emotion in order to believe the logical part. The father left the mother, or vice versa, because the marriage failed, never because of a child's inability to play counsellor or to prevent a punch from being swung.

The childhood environment can be made negative and hostile when children have to listen to the parents blaming each other for the breakdown. After separation and the visits to the two parents, the child becomes a pawn in a battle of blame. The father might blame the mother and will tell stories that put him in the right and the mother at fault. Or this can happen the other way around. Come what may, the child is used as a go-between or as an audience that has to be won over for support.

You will see the children after they have grown up. They will carry the debris from a war that was never theirs.

Attitudes.
Clients might have attitudes that they have 'inherited' from parents. Such things as bigotry, racism, homophobia and so on. Clients have to be able to make a decision for themselves rather than adopting somebody else's view. Again, the role of the therapist in changing social values must be questioned. If you lecture the client on being more accepting of 'proper' views, you are taking on a different role. Are your views judgemental? Are you correcting things that are beyond your brief as a therapist? You might just be reflecting the

147

dictatorial style of a parent who caused a problem in the first place.

Sometimes a child can blame him/herself for not being good enough. Standards are set, rules must be obeyed and the child is criticised because of failure to meet the levels set. This then reflects in the child's low self-esteem. This is something that continues into adulthood. A client needs to accept their achievements and ignore the criticism from the past. Sometimes parents are in competition with relatives and/or friends about the achievements of their children. They feel that the achievements of their children reflect their abilities to raise and teach their offspring in a way that demonstrates their hidden skills and intelligence.

Some children develop later than others. Some will reach their own ceiling that is lower than has been set. Some children will rebel against the pressure and will refuse to do any work so that the parent's commands will have the opposite effect to that desired.

Abusive parents
See the chapter on abuse.

Step parents
When a lion becomes too old to keep his territory and his mate, a new male will move in. That new male will kill any cubs that are left. The new male has no interest in protecting another lion's offspring.

When a step parent moves into a family adjustments will be made. A step parent might feel in competition with the person they have replaced. A step child is in competition with step-siblings. In short, the dynamics of the family will have changed. A step parent might seem to favour their own biological offspring against what might be seen as an added expense in their life.

This will have consequences for the child or children that will be needed to be sorted when they arrive as clients. They might have lost self-esteem through jealousy or through rivalry. They even feel that the parent loves the new partner more than them and that they were made to feel that they were nothing more than a nuisance.

The role of the therapist is to develop a new perspective for the client to view the situation that caused their problem.

Death of parents/siblings/children.
The death of individuals who are close to the client will change their views. Parental death will open guilt for things said and not said.

Sibling deaths, particularly the death of a twin will open up relief that it was somebody else that died with, ironically, a huge amount of guilt because it was somebody else who died.

You have to ask yourself if you are competent to be a bereavement counsellor. If you see your role as a therapist in a different light, then it is the time when you should refer a client to a specialist in the area of death.

Past, Present and Future

A lot of people go through life like they are rowing a boat. They look at where they have been (the PAST) rather than where they are going (the FUTURE). Unknown Source

It makes a great deal of sense to me that we, as therapists, should help the client to look at the past and sieve out the bad bits. However, those pieces should be discarded leaving the better memories to work as a foundation for the present and future. The past is important but if we keep looking at it as if looking perpetually in the rear-view mirror when driving, we will crash. An occasional glimpse behind, suffices. The important thing to do is look at the future as if it is a clear and clean road.

Problems have to be dealt with in order to move forward but there is a point when the problem has to be considered to be something that the client **had**. This means that the desired outcome exists in the present.

Affirmations work because they recognise a future desire in the present tense! This strange paradox works. When a client arrives for therapy they carry their problem with them as if it were a huge part of their very being. One powerful way to bring about change is to develop positive affirmations. These have to be set in the present tense because a change that will happen means that the status quo still presides over the current situation.

They want a release from their problems and an affirmation will work **after** they have dealt with the causes of the problem. The way in which people think and act can be changed by encouraging the client to define new goals rather than living out old frames of being.

"I will become positive" is weak against, "I am positive" because it still affirms the negativity with which the clients present themselves.

If I say to a client 'you will get better' and use that as a suggestion or affirmation then I am implying that the client still has the problem. If I get the client to say that the problem is something that they had, but now they are free of whatever that problem was, they have a positive affirmation of a new state.

To use verbal pictures, they have to uncouple the railway carriage that carried their problem and let it glide into a siding so that the train can move forward unencumbered.

Alternatively, if they have an old car that is troublesome, it is never enough to assure them that one day they will get a new one. They have to acknowledge that they had and old car, but now, they have a new one.

The past is where the problem started. The past is what influences the present. When the present time is seen as being fixed to the past then the problem remains.

Past problem influences future as it is still attached			
	Past problem	**Present**	**Future is hard because the past is still attached**

Past left behind gives good future		
	Past problems left behind	**Present**	**Future good**

When the future is fixed to the present time and a gap is made then the past has been separated. This enables the client to move forward unencumbered by the past.

151

Phobias

The thing I fear most is fear.
Michel Eyquem de Montaigne (1533-1592) French philosopher.

A phobia is a condition rather than a specific response (the phobic response is panic). With a phobia there is an irrational fear of an object or situation. As the response of a panic attack may be triggered by actual exposure to that object or situation, or may be manifested by the mere thought of it, the coping mechanism that is often used is that of avoidance.

Phobic stimuli include a variety of things or situations such as crowds (e.g. shopping, speech making), social situations (e.g. being exposed to the judgements of others at parties), animals (e.g. snakes, spiders, sharks), inanimate objects (e.g. bridges), natural occurrences (thunder and lightning), illness, blood (or perhaps the circumstances in which blood is seen).

It is difficult to reason that there is any other cause of a phobic reaction than that of conditioning, as babies and small children are usually born phobia free. It is reasonable to assume that a fear response is something which we are pre-disposed to have for survival, for example the atavistic phobias, described above, involving snakes, spiders, lizards and other life threatening situations in our primeval days. Crowds of strangers could have been, and might still be, hostile.

It is pertinent to note that phobias elicit a strong survival response, that of flight-or-flight.

However, such a reaction that is much stronger than is necessary is debilitating in our safer times, as is the response to inappropriate objects or situations. This perhaps gives a better clue to the causes of phobias. What might seem inappropriate to the conscious mind might seem very appropriate to the unconscious mind through misconstrued associations.

With all examples of phobias it is reasonable to understand that cause and effect sometimes have a cryptic connection to the need to survive, but the encryption can sometimes make the phobic response seem out of reach. The response, therefore, cannot be eliminated because the true cause is unrecognised, and therefore cannot be mitigated. The job of the therapist is to find, and deal with, the real cause.

When you are treating phobias, treat the problem that you and your client understand!

A Latin word for whatever it is with phobia tagged on the end means nothing to your client. Arachnophobia is a fear of spiders. What you are treating is the client's fear of spiders and that they understand. After talking in Latin then the next time a client sees an 'arachnid' and is happy, then you will feel you have achieved success. However, the client never sees a spider as an arachnid but as spider. You will have failed.

Latin never makes you seem more intelligent, it interferes with communication. A more pertinent example is agoraphobia. It is often understood as a fear of open spaces. However the word agora is Latin for market place and the fear is about being in a situation where escape might be difficult, physically or emotionally. So if a client tells you that they suffer from agoraphobia and you treat them for a fear of open spaces, you have got it wrong! Treat what you <u>both</u> understand to be the issue.

Without going into hundreds of pages about each phobia, we can get to the root cause of each one in a general way for the sake of efficiency. The fight-or-flight response protects us in a basic way. When something is perceived to be a threat, we are urged to avoid it.

There are phobias caused by bad experiences. These might be in car crashes, dark alleys, abuse and so on. A fear of seeing or being sick is quite common. One of the things the clients have in common is that they have rarely seen or been sick. The other thing is a huge fear about even talking about it.

Then there are phobias related to a reaction to an unknown cause. The client might feel uncomfortable and fearful in situations that appear to have nothing to link them.

To deal with a phobia look for a root cause and the emotional connections. A spider phobic was probably frightened by a screaming mother rather than a spider but displaced the fear caused onto the spider rather than mother. There is more about atavistic phobias under that heading.

Think of phobias as panic attacks that have a direct cause from a specific stimulus. You have to find the basis of that cause and then change the reaction to one of wary acceptance rather than escape by dramatic means. This is important. If we take a person with a fear of heights to the release of the problem to such an extent that they happily get very close to the edges of cliffs, we would be irresponsible to say the least. Flying phobics should be able to enjoy flying rather than cope with it. A snake phobic should never feel the urge to kiss a puff-adder!

A change of attitude is essential. The phobic stimulus has to be seen in a different light, that of <u>little</u> potential harm rather than being life-threatening.

Public Speaking

Drawing is speaking to the eye; talking is painting to the ear.
Joseph Joubert (1754-1824) French moralist.

The elements than cause anxiety with public speakers need to be exposed and corrected. Not everybody is a natural extrovert, and at the same time, not everybody who is shy in front of an audience is a dyed-in-the-wool introvert.

The cause of the client's reluctance to perform in public should be discovered and dealt with. This could be from dominating and/or critical parents. Perhaps it came from having to speak at school in front of a disparaging teacher or bullying classmates. It might have come later in life at University or in a work situation. This means that you should also establish what the talk or speech that has prompted the client to visit you is going to be. Some people are in control in front of a small audience but panic in front of a larger one. Some are fine when sitting but unhappy when on their feet.

Public speaking is an anxiety creating situation and as such can be a major fear or even phobia. (I use the distinction in the context of performing but hating it and as a phobic the solution is avoidance.) Your task is twofold. First of all, deal with the root of anxiety as a cause in order to reduce or eliminate it. Secondly coach the client in relaxation and presentation techniques.

People with a fear of public speaking will have lots of things in common. The fight or flight response is in full flow. They will speak softly. They will speak quickly and be short of breath. They forget their words. They will be frozen in a static position yet they want to run away.

When the clients have released their anxiety I like to ask them to stand up in my office and read a short passage from a book. They will demonstrate the problem quite clearly, and they will probably fail to understand what they have just read. Like a stone skimming over the surface of the waves, the contact with the main body of the work is lost to the client and to the audience.

You then become a constructive coach.

The client should read the passage again but this time taking a diaphragmatic breath on each piece of punctuation. A slow and gentle breath for a comma and a deeper one for a full stop. The pauses in the reading add depth to what is being read and it slows the delivery.

Get them to use their hands to draw pictures about the contents. A huge amount of communication is non-verbal. Think back 50,000 years. If a black mamba was moving across a path we never had the vocabulary to say, 'Excuse me, old chap. There is a highly venomous snake just in front of you. Take extra care to avoid treading on it.'

We would have pointed, hissed and imitated wriggling and biting using our arms and hands. No words would have been used but the message would have been received in no uncertain terms.

You can demonstrate the point by asking the client to describe the last holiday that they went on. They will talk about a beach or a city but you will be unable to see it. When you ask them questions about what it looked like, and you ask them to use their hands, they will see the scene more vividly and so will you.

Remember examples such as Marcel Marceau and his ability to mime. Think of a ventriloquist's dummy. It has to move in order to give a stronger message than being stuck on a pole in the middle of the stage, frozen in a pose!

There is another benefit to being animated that you can demonstrate. When the arms are raised then the diaphragm is more used than when the arms are held stiffly by the side.

The client should be encouraged to 'break the ice' with the audience.

Once he/she has said a few words before the presentation then the inertia that could be felt at the start of the presentation is overcome. The client's mind feels that the first obstacle has been broken down.

Some sort of eye contact helps. This might be with nobody in particular but a slow look to the left, then the right and then the middle of the audience extends the depth of the presentation or speech. It makes it seem more personal to each member of the audience. Even if the presentation is being made with slides and the room is dark, the audience will pick up the head movement.

The client should understand the audience's needs. They are there, perhaps to learn. The client has been asked to speak because that person knows something that the audience would like to know. Perhaps a best-man is talking about the groom. Here there is a sympathetic and friendly audience who are rooting for the speechmaker. And so on. Every audience is sympathetic and friendly, no matter what. They will <u>never</u> be the critical people who caused the problem in the first place.

The client should practice their talk over and over when they are at home. They should slow down, paint the images with their hands and work on breathing at the right time. They should employ an imaginary Constructive Coach, who is an inner voice that praises and picks up on little details where there could be an improvement. This inner voice is always positive. It is the opposite in every way to the original critic who knocked the client's confidence for no good reason.

CHECKLIST

Resolve the cause of the anxiety.
- Find the causes and resolve them in the current time frame.
- Look for reinforcing occasions where the client felt bad.
- Put experiences into a time frame. The nervousness of a thirteen year old talking in Assembly about something that is misunderstood has to change when that person is a thirty year old employee giving a talk about his/her area of expertise. Yet

if the previous situation dominates the emotion of fear then the idea of relaxing is far away.

Technique practice:
- Slow the delivery down.
- Use of the diaphragm.
- Use of the hands by the speaker to describe what is being said.
- Animation of the speaker.
- Break the ice before speaking.
- Make eye contact with a few people to extend the involvement.
- The client should understand what the audience's needs are.
- Let the client rehearse in front of you as the Constructive Coach.
- Show the client how to practice using an imaginary Constructive Coach.

Relationship Splits

'If I Could Turn Back the Hands of Time.' R. Kelly song.

'I will change. I will never do it again. I do love you' and so on.

These are some of the words that are spoken by your clients to their partners before they come to see you. They are looking for magic! The client hopes that by seeing a therapist the problem will be resolved with a third party.

Sometimes those words are meant as an intention, other times they are said as a stalling mechanism for a failing relationship. You should be able to differentiate between the two extremes.

With the first type, problems within a person can be dealt with and resolved but you are never able to fix the consequences. If an angry client lashes out then the promise to change might be honest and you can help. The thing you are unable to do is offer to persuade the wronged partner that the angry person has changed for good. You can never be part of the promise that the problem has been resolved to ensure the safety of the hurt party. Never confuse the two issues. Your job would be to treat anger rather than act as a relationship guidance counsellor. This would be an extra brief, to be treated in a different way, if you are qualified by experience to do so.

The second type is asking for a respite rather than help. Hoping that time, and your apparent help will restore the status quo you should be under no illusion that you are helping nothing but a stall. The reactions or the client will tell you which scenario you have. A highly co-operative and open client who shows genuine remorse will feature with the first type.

An arrogance and lack of co-operation will signal the second. You should decide to be very wary of the second type. You should be conscious of the dangers that you could cause. Question that type of client deeply to find out what their real motives are for seeking help.

Then, if necessary, explain fully that you can only help people who are genuine in their search for treatment and do your absolute utmost to turn the client to the direction of a happy future with the problem resolved in depth. Everybody should seek happiness but to do so they have to admit that they are the cause of upset and that only by change will they find it rather than set up a smokescreen that will hide their behaviour for a while until the smoke clears. Then the original problem will, once again, raise its ugly head.

Reject before being rejected.
There is another phenomenon that you will encounter. I refer to this as 'reject before you are rejected'. This is a self-esteem issue whereby the client will be lonely because he/she is without friends. They will have been hurt in the past and they adopt the strategy of never committing fully to a new relationship in case they are hurt again. Thus they will push a new friend or suitor away when the relationship develops to the point where the client feels vulnerable.

The rescue comes from building the client's self-esteem to where they can become able to take the risk of rejection happening. It becomes a 'win/lose but be happy' situation rather than a 'lose/lose result come what may'. Find the cause of the feelings of rejection and build confidence. If a parent or a boy/girlfriend was the cause then other people they have yet to meet will be different. Their acceptance of the rejected client will have a totally different foundation.

Ownership
Sometimes after a relationship has ended one of the two people will claim ownership of the other party. If one person leaves a house they will want to keep a key to enter the house whenever they want. The excuse might be access to children or to a toolkit. This, of course makes new relationships difficult, if not impossible. That is why the partner who has left will do it. They are jealous and possessive. They want their cake and they want to eat it as well.

Your client has to gain enough confidence to change the locks, take a Court injunction or other action to stop it. You will never tell a client to do this, your job is to help the client to be strong enough to do it of their own accord. Your advice is never to be given.

Needless to say, the partner in a relationship that has been ended by another person will have feelings of depression. This is because they have lost somebody that they wanted. There is a loss of hope in restoring the relationship and of ever having another that is successful. They will blame themselves and search for reasons. This process will drag up every dark thought in their psyches. The hope that you can give is that things will get better, life goes on. The client has to be able to prepare for, and accept change.

Secondary Gains

Secondary gains are strange phenomena. Clients can develop symptoms of problems to avoid what is thought of as a primary issue. An example of this might be excessive weight gain to make the client less attractive to a partner in order to avoid sexual advances which caused the original problems in the client's life.

Another example might be exhibiting symptoms and feelings of stress to avoid having to work with a bullying boss or threatening workmates.

It might be to gain sympathy from a partner or parent during a poor relationship by showing as a headache.

Clients might present with symptoms of a problem that you will start to see as secondary gain. Rather than dismissing them as hypochondriacs, treat the real cause of their problems. In the first example treat the abuse that happened many years ago. In the second enable the client to deal with the stress and/or build enough confidence to look for alternative employment. In the third example the treatment should be for the reasons as to why the relationship is going through troubled times.

It is something to look for with smokers. Ask if the partner smokes and if so, where <u>did</u> the two people smoke. If it was together in the garden perhaps it was the only time that they talked. If this is the situation, the client must arrange a different reason to talk to the 'other-half'. You need to take away any excuse to start again.

Sexual Problems

The sexual problems that you will encounter will include premature ejaculation, failure to ejaculate and erectile failure for men. Women will see you frigidity, vaginismus and promiscuity.

Physical causes must be checked by a medical practitioner before you go ahead with therapy. Some symptoms could point to prostate problems; others to high blood pressure and so on. Some be caused by sexually transmitted illnesses. So unless you are a medical practitioner as well as a therapist, the client has to seek medical advice before undertaking therapy.

Smoking and drinking can affect performance. Smoking reduces blood flow. Excessive drinking of alcohol will have devastating results for a man's sexual life.

These can be the first course of action. The client needs to stop either, or both, activities. You should treat the cause before you can resolve the problem.

If your client leads a sober and tobacco free life and is free of any other physical problem then you look for lifestyle problems such as stress or relationship issues. For males and females the underlying wish to avoid pregnancy will change their attitudes towards intercourse. A woman could become unwilling to have sex and be seen as frigid. A man might fail to reach orgasm for fear of making his partner pregnant.

All of that said, the psychological roots of sexual problems can be with our old friend, or enemy, the fight-or-flight response. In order for a man to ejaculate, the sympathetic branch has to kick in. The orgasm will be the result of a sudden change to where the heart rate rises as the result of adrenaline being released. This is in contrast to the situation where the parasympathetic branch needs to be working to relax a man enough to enable his erection.

P is for parasympathetic, or point.
S is for sympathetic, or shoot. You can remember it that way.

If a man has erectile failure, is he relaxed enough during love making? Perhaps this will relate to bad experiences in his past when he was caught in a compromising situation or when he felt overpowered by a woman's advances and demands through his inexperience or naivety.

Premature ejaculation can come from anxiety. In our primeval past the main objective of sex was to have pleasure and as a result, perhaps impregnate a mate. Think of a sexual act. The man is vulnerable. In whichever position he adopts he will have his back to unknown dangers or if the woman is on top he will be like a tortoise on its back and unable to respond to threat easily. It made sense to ejaculate quickly and be aware of surroundings.

Now that we make love in safe places in the main (although some people are stimulated by making love in dangerous or exposed places) that sense of being able to hold on to pleasure and to enable the female partner to receive pleasure has grown. It has become an issue of mutual satisfaction so you can enable the client to feel safe and secure in a relationship and allow him to relax enough to maintain his parasympathetic state and thus delay his orgasm. Worrying about premature ejaculation often adds the anxiety to the situation that makes it happen because the sympathetic branch kicks in. Your client can play games by double bluffing the system. When he 'tries' to ejaculate and makes it a pressure to do so, often the 'desired' result fails to happen. This works because it is a negative suggestion and distracts the mind from worrying about one outcome with another.

The above applies equally to impotence. A man will need to feel safe and secure in his relationship as well as his location. A partner should be sympathetic where possible and encourage trust and support.

Some clients can be affected by watching pornography. The man will be set impossible standards of longevity and female arousal. Failure is never an option. The stud will be large in his private parts and the insatiable female can always be satisfied. If the scenarios are believed then the bar is set too high and stress and pressure to perform as well as the porn-star will be enough to ensure that the man never performs at all. The other issue is that the man will often be only able to achieve an erection and orgasm if he masturbates. This signals that he is able to perform the sexual act when he is alone and safe. There is nothing wrong with his body but his mindset needs to be sorted out.

Remember that performers in porn films are helped by Viagra and editing. They are fictional and documentaries show that they are never happy with their lives. Difficult situations that are dirty and unhappy rule their lives. They do it to make a living and rarely because they enjoy the pure sexual act as a demonstration of a loving relationship.

Your clients should know that there is a difference between fiction and real life.

For women, the causes of problems are manifold. Bad experiences, abuse and so on will have an effect. You need history and analysis to help you to help them. Another cause can be guilt. See the section on sexual abuse, above.

Siblings

**It snowed last year too: I made a snowman and my brother knocked
it down and I knocked my brother down and then we had tea.**
~Dylan Thomas

Wildlife documentaries show us that young creatures fight and
squabble in order to train their bodies and skills for their lives as
adults. When young they have to compete for attention and therefore
food from their mothers. The runt of the litter is weak and the chances
of survival are diminished.

Humans are animals. Never forget that. Yet we can communicate with
words as well as actions so our fighting and squabbling is verbal as
well as physical. People fight for attention. We fight for the right to
dominate siblings. We fight to be perceived as different and special.

This can show as clients who are fussy eaters because they have
control over the meal table. The mother has to cook an individual meal
for a fussy eater who, by this tactic, gets more attention. When treating
fussy eaters, by the way, emphasise that after a childhood and young
adulthood of gaining attention by refusing to eat what other members
of the family eat, the mother, and perhaps now, the partner, is irritated
by the behaviour. The need now is for the client to eat whatever is
offered to gain new attention by people praising the change. This
works!

In common with other creatures, as a species we fight when young.
We are hard-wired to dislike the competition. Also, brothers should
dislike sisters and vice versa in order to prevent inter-breeding. This
rivalry changes when the siblings reach maturity as the brother, now
the primeval male, becomes protective of his 'weaker' sister. In our
modern lives girls/women fight as well as men, but the drive remains.

This is probably the same instinctive drive that seems to make fathers
love their daughters more than their sons and mothers love sons more

than daughters. Rather than being sexual in motive this is for protection and nurture. Fathers are wary of boyfriends. They know what men are after! They want their daughters to have responsible and protective mates/partners rather than 'predators'.

Mothers want sons to be strong and well cared for so that they can become successful hunters, albeit for money rather than game these days. Also, in primeval tribal societies, the sons would have a drive to protect their mothers if anything happened to the fathers.

The rivalry between siblings is very often an act rather than real hatred. When young siblings grow they will become protective of each other in fraught situations. However the facade will remain in day to day life. It can become real in situations such as sharing the inheritances from the death of a parent. These scars will run deep and will last for a very long time.

Where there can be real dislike is when step and ½ siblings are involved. One of the parents that a client lives, or has lived, with is a birth parent and the other is an added parent. The children will have a drive to diminish the presence of an acquired sibling. The dislike can become a real hatred. Step and ½ siblings can lie about the competition to gain the high ground and this leads to major problems for your clients.

Siblings, especially in big numbers, will fight for the control of speech. When they do this they can develop the practice of speaking in long sentences with short, sharp intakes of breath in order to prevent being interrupted. This causes the high-chested style of breathing that leads to anxiety. Usually the younger siblings will acquire this debilitating habit. It is something to be considered with clients who suffer from anxiety and panic. It can start around the meal table when there is competition for attention.

Smokers

The best way to stop smoking is to carry wet matches.
Unknown Source

There are two schools of thought about smoking. One says that nicotine is a highly addictive drug, as addictive as heroin and cocaine according to the Royal College of Physicians in 2000. The other says smoking is a habit that needs to be broken, like finger nail biting.

My view is that, without dismissing the main theories, there is another perceived benefit from smoking, that is, it encourages smokers to breathe correctly although at a very high price!

Before you throw this book down in disgust at that comment, this is the way in which I conduct most Stop Smoking sessions.

Say to the client, 'I will phrase this question in a strange way because you are now a non-smoker. You have walked through my door. How many cigarettes DID you smoke per day?' I want them to believe that they have come to see me for a Stop Smoking session because they want to be non smokers!

After the client gives you their details about how many cigarettes per day they smoked, and when they have given the age at which they started, ask him/her to take a deep breath. They will invariably inflate the chest, tighten the neck and stomach muscles and they will look very uncomfortable. Then ask the smoker to put the left hand, if they are right-handed, on the stomach and the other hand on the high chest. Reverse the hands if they are left handed. Ask them to breathe in to push the hand on the stomach out with their breath whilst keeping the chest still. You will notice that the chest inflates again and the hand on the stomach will remain still or will actually move in.

Then ask the smoker to imagine that they are taking a 'drag' or 'draw' on a cigarette whilst holding the other hand on the stomach. Now you, and they, will notice that the hand on the stomach moves out!

You should demonstrate to the client that we are conditioned, unwittingly, from childhood by teachers and parents into breathing with the upper chest. Tell the client that there are three words that everybody will respond to. Ask if they would like to know what those words are and when they say 'yes', inform them that you will tell them in a while. Then say, with a tone of authority, 'Sit up straight.'

Watch the client spring up into an upright position. Some will even apologise. Tell the client that they are the words and make your apology as well. Say that you have no right to tell them how to sit and ask them to relax. You have made the point.

We are taught to hold ourselves upright by a continual bombardment from culture. Fashion and the media show us big chested men and women with flat stomachs as the desired norm. Children from the early school days are encouraged to hold themselves to look like stars. Then puberty comes along and the pressure continues. You will find that most of your smoking clients started to smoke between the ages of 10 to 13 and the cause will be peer pressure.

There is an interesting point about the starting age. You can work out how long they have been smoking and explain that addictive things have one thing in common. The longer a person uses an addictive product then the more of it has to be used each day to get the same effect. Thus an alcoholic starts with a glass of sherry per day and goes to a bottle or two of vodka. A heroin addict will increase its use to the point where they can overdose. A smoker will maintain the habit at the same number of cigarettes per day for many years. Is this a sign of a true addiction to nicotine?

I teach my smoking clients how to breathe using their diaphragms. I show them how to do the 4 x 4 exercise, described later, and ask them to do it twice a day for life. I show them how to breathe correctly when they are sitting. I explain that pets and young children should be role models for correct breathing practice.

Then I start the 'stop smoking' session. This contains suggestions for improvement in health, smell (as in having a better sense of smell as well as personal hygiene) and feeling better. Tobacco smoke contains more than 4200 chemicals of which over 2000 are toxic including cyanide, arsenic, carbon monoxide, formaldehyde, acetone and polonium 210.

If the smoker has children, talk about 'smell memory'. Every parent will remember the smell of their new born child. This is part of bonding. They will remember with fond emotions the aromas of after-shaves or perfumes of first loves. Therefore explain that their children will associate the smell of tobacco smoke on the clothes of parents with the love that is shared. This means that the children or grandchildren of smokers will develop positive attitudes towards the smell of smoke and will be more likely to start. This is emotional blackmail that is aimed at saving lives.

All suggestions for stopping smoking must be positive. I have seen scripts that talk about 'if you carry on smoking you will die' and 'imagine yourself standing next to your grave watching your loved-ones crying.' You will never have a 100% success rate with smokers so if you use suggestions of death then the clients who start to smoke after you have seen them will be carrying what amounts to a voodoo curse.

Your clients need positive reasons to stop. Negativity has failed the client because every cigarette packet they have bought explains the dangers yet they have come to see you for help.

Affirm the new way in which to breathe. Affirm the health benefits but in personal terms such as being more attractive to their partners.

There is a part of my sessions in which I require the client's participation. I will ask them to imagine a time-scale going back to their young childhood. Then I will ask them to move forward to see the point at which they had their first smoke. Then I will ask them to ask to that younger version of him/herself why they are starting to smoke. Then I want them to explain to that person why they are wrong in starting to smoke and how they would benefit from being a non-smoker. Rather than admonishing the younger person, the client is supporting a decision to stop. Part of this is the client internally acknowledging that they want and need to stop. Sometimes the client will become emotional and let tears go. Then I will ask the client to hear the younger person ask when the time will come when the client will stop and the answer is always the day of the session. Then I ask the client to hear the younger version say how proud he/she is that the client is now a non-smoker, and then ask the client to say to him/herself how proud they are.

All of this is done with the client thinking, rather than talking out loud, through the dialogue with their younger self. They will signal completion to you at the end of each bit by raising a finger.

Give as many positive suggestions and affirmations as possible and remind the ex-smoker about breathing.

I then ask the client to imagine how they will be in one year after the session. They imagine how fresh they smell and how good they look. To help to eliminate worries about weight gain they should see themselves at a good shape.

I give a CD to each client and ask them to listen to it once per day for the first three days after the session and then every-other day for three more times. There is a magical number in communication and that number is seven. People will be better affected after something is said seven times. The CD I give is my recording and it has the session content on it but it is stated in the past tense. In other words, if during the session I say 'you will be amazed at how easily you now stop smoking', the CD says 'you are amazed at how easily you stopped smoking'. My CD also contains a relaxation and motivational track to make it worth keeping. If a client gives the CD to a friend then it is unavailable if the client needs future reinforcement. The instructions for breathing are repeated on the cover.

If a client asks you what happens if they start to smoke after your treatment, refuse to acknowledge the possibility of failure. Therapists who offer a free or half price session if the first session fails to work are making a huge suggestion that the treatment has a low chance of success. You and the client must be confident about their success.

I ask the, now, ex-smoker if they would like me to crush any cigarettes that they have with them. Most will relish the idea. The habitual part of smoking is strong. If something happens that would have made the client reach for a cigarette then habit will kick in if cigarettes are available.

The new habit has to be that of taking diaphragmatic breaths instead of lighting up in times of stress. When the old habit of reaching for a cigarette is disabled then the new habit of breathing for a healthy life has a much better chance of becoming established.

Stress

The components of anxiety, stress, fear, and anger do not exist independently of you in the world. They simply do not exist in the physical world, even though we talk about them as if they do.
Wayne Dyer (1940-?) American psychotherapist, author and lecturer.

STRESS

Stress is an umbrella word. Therefore, it has many meanings which depend very much on the context in which it is used. For example, it can be:

- A short-term reaction to specific events.
- A long-term reaction.
- Something that results from situational problems such as work, social or domestic pressures.
- Something that results from a series of negative events such as a succession of accidents.
- The result of ill health.
- The pre-cursor to other problems.

Perhaps the linking meaning is in the individual's ability to cope with the situation he/she is in. There is a link to the psychological input of the perception of threat mentioned above. For example, the term positive stress is often used in a motivational sense where a choice can be made. The stress caused by the approach in time to a parachute jump can be controlled by cancelling it after it is booked and paid for, and it is likely to be felt as excitement. However, the stress in the same situation by an Army recruit is less controllable, and is likely to be felt as negative stress, having powerful physical and emotional effects.

It is never just to do with overload of work or problems. Stress from boredom amongst the unemployed is just as debilitating as stress caused by long work hours.

I like the definition of the causes of misery (stress?) as "wanting things that you can't have, and having things that you don't want".

People who believe that they have control of their own lives have less stress than those who believe that they are victims of circumstance. This suggests that there is a large internal (psychological) input into the susceptibility that an individual has to stress, rather than to the external situation as such.

It seems that the essence of stress is the inability to cope and the inability to control. It can be seen as part of the fight-or-flight response over a much longer period of time. This makes it much more insidious in that its effects are cumulative and move toward a crisis point.

Moreover, stress can be linked with anger, suppressed or expressed. This connects it more to the 'fight' part of the 'fight-or-flight' response. Anger rarely brings positive results; an employee might want to punch his/her boss, but suppresses the urge for material security. Instead, this impulse to fight the boss is satisfied by verbal or physical fights with his/her partner. The inability to fight unemployment and boredom is expressed as anger with the situation, society etc. Perhaps 'road rage' and 'baby bashing' are the physical realisations of stress.

It is as if stress is about sustained, suppressed anger, the restrained fight response which sometimes erupts into attack, whereas panic and phobias are about fear, running away from the threat.

The causes of stress are diverse. Although it can be considered to be just one disorder for the sake of generalised communication, the causes, and indeed the pre-dispositions to stress, are as numerous as the number of people who suffer from it.

Thus, within a family, two brothers can have the same type of upbringing, the same career, but one becomes stressed and the other does not. Perhaps sibling rivalry has a bearing in this situation. Perhaps an overbearing boss reminds a sufferer of an authoritarian father. Perhaps an over-careful mother causes anxiety when she nags her son to make sure his underpants are clean in case he has an accident, which is brought to the surface by his traffic-jam beset journey to work everyday. In short, there are numerous causes of stress, which are very different in nature, but similar in the effect of causing deep-seated worry later in life when adjacent pressures are felt.

The feelings of stress will manifest themselves in different ways; the reactions to the feelings of unease will vary. To use an analogy, stress is like an egg-timer, with the various causes at the top, the various reactions at the bottom, and the constricted part is the generalised description of 'stress', and this common denominator is the individual's ability to cope with the circumstances of his life.

The effect of stress, the sustained fight or flight response, is the physiological damage caused. This shows as:

- Heart disease and high blood pressure from increased heart rate.
- Digestive system problems because blood flow is reduced and the digestion process is slowed or delayed.
- Skin problems from reduced blood flow.
- Headaches and migraines from physical and cognitive changes.
- Increased frequency of urination.
- Breathing changes causing hyperventilation.
- Impotence and loss of sexual drive.
- Weakening of the immune response.

There are also psychological problems including:

- Loss of a sense of humour.
- Mood and emotional change.
- Depression from feeling helpless.

TREATMENT

It is necessary to find two major components of the client's problem; the reasons for their predisposition to stress, and the circumstances that are causing stress at the current time. This involves analysis followed by a more direct questioning. When the factors in the client's earlier life are exposed and dealt with then the therapist should concentrate on how those events have influenced the present situation. A process of reframing prior events will take place to ensure that the client has a better perspective of life pressures and how they can be handled.

Once again, the issue of control comes to the fore. If the client is controlled by another person or circumstances then they must gain a sense of control for their own lives. When a person feels that they have control then they feel less stressed because they have more influence over events.

When somebody feels that they have little control then they will be stressed by the demands of others.

It is also important that the client learns coping techniques that will cover everything from anger control to relaxation.

Weight

There is a joke about a two page diet book giving a system that works. On page one it says, 'Eat less, and take more exercise'. On page two it says, 'See page one!'

WEIGHT CONTROL THERAPIES

In simple terms, you will see four types of people who want to lose weight.

1. Those who want to lose between 1 to 3 stones. (14 to 42 pounds or 6 to 19 kilos.)
2. Those who want, and need, to lose substantially more and who are obese.
3. Those who have been told to lose weight by somebody in authority such as a dance instructor.
4. Those who want to lose weight because they have an eating disorder.

I will deal with each type one at a time.

Those who want to lose between 1 to 3 stones. (14 to 42 pounds or 6 to 19 kilos.) Please Note: This first part for a small amount of weight loss is adapted and abridged from The Secret Language of Hypnotherapy.

This is done as suggestion therapy and I back it up with a CD recording. This CD contains a different session to the one given for the reasons explained later. It also explains the structure of weight loss system and adds a relaxation track which is a metaphor for changes in perception of achievement. This is to motivate the client to keep on going with the programme.

The therapist should become familiar with the following and then give a précis to the client as a pre-amble to the hypnosis session. This is a different method and the therapist has to explain it in order for it to have any credibility in a world where people can only look to dieting

177

and calorie counting for help other than having radical surgery.

People in the Western world are under huge body-image stress. Our ideals of looking good are imposed by movie makers and media superstars. We are bombarded by images of people on television, in films and magazines.

Career progression seems to be related to personal appearance. Fashionable clothes and fashionable body shapes are highly valued, highly prized and often highly priced. People feel that they need to look good to succeed in the giant business corporations of the world.

Children are persuaded to look and act as young adults. They are given role models who are pop-stars and super-models. They are the celebrities who follow the ideas that they need to 'look good' to be successful. Sadly, this usually translates as being thin and sexy. Youngsters attend schools that are the meeting places for youth. They are also crucibles for ideals and criticisms. Unfortunately, they can also be the high-pressure boiler houses where peer pressure and bullying take place.

Set against the huge marketing effort for high energy foods and drinks, items that are often high in sugar and fat, the drive to be thin is enormous and difficult. Those who 'succeed' too well risk eating disorders such as anorexia and bulimia. Those who 'fail' can be seduced into obesity. We have been fed a rich diet of the perfect body shape.

The following method for weight control has nothing to do with dieting or calorie counting. It has nothing to do with fads such as elimination diets, nor eating only protein or carbohydrates or high fibre foods. Those methods can be antagonistic to the natural shape control systems that we have and often end up with the opposite results to those you intended.

We have body images, blueprints or what are called 'set weights', a biological term used for animals whose weights or shapes only change through starvation if food supplies run out.

Note. Most of the references are made for women. Of the thousands of people that I have helped to lose weight, most have been female. Therefore I am not being sexist in any way. I am simply making the narrative easier to use. The method works equally well for men.

Through homeostasis, described above, body shapes are maintained within a small range. If we can imagine that we possess a 'blue-print' for shape, then it helps. To use computer terms, we can accept that we possess a 'virtual' thermometer for our temperature, and a virtual chemical laboratory for hormones. To advance the idea of a 'virtual' body-shape-blueprint is reasonable.

Those 'blue-prints' keep our shapes the same, give-or-take a few pounds, until interfered with by life circumstances, social influences and by our attempts to consciously lose weight by starvation methods. Obsessive calorie counting and rapid diets antagonise our well adjusted systems.

This maintenance of our bodily systems takes place in a small part of the brain called the hypothalamus. This brain structure, roughly the size of a walnut, receives sensory information from the body. It then regulates the body to ensure stability.

Metabolism is the name for the chemical reactions that take place in the body that use nutrients to provide energy and to make, or replace, body materials. Metabolism increases during pregnancy, menstruation and the consumption of food. It also speeds up during activity and when there are excess thyroid hormones. It decreases as we get older and during starvation.

The hypothalamus is involved in metabolism. It has affects on levels of hormones such as insulin, thyroxin and leptin. Leptin, from the Greek *leptos* meaning thin, was discovered as recently as 1994 and relates to the fat mass of the body.

These hormones, and others, are associated with appetite, weight control and metabolism. They are all involved with fat mass and body weight, something referred to as 'set-weight' for all animals, strangely, with the exception of humans. It is the ideal weight, or shape, for each individual. All creatures have internal body images that are established and regulated. You can watch 100,000 wildebeests run through an African plain and they all look the same. Nobody has interfered with their ideas about fashionable shapes.

Of course, we humans are animals. We also have 'set weights' but I will refer to them as the body-shape-blueprint as we need to develop a conscious awareness of our body shapes.

The term, weight, is measured in pounds and kilos. They are artificial concepts that have little relevance to our understanding of our body shapes. To demonstrate this point, if you weigh yourself in pounds, convert that number to stones or kilograms, these new numbers mean very little to you.

Our blueprints have been inherited from our primeval ancestors, but we like to think that we can eradicate our natures with conscious resolve. Our awareness of our shapes is at the root of our weight problems. We interfere with our outer appearances to the detriment of our inherent systems. Rather than dieting or calorie counting we need to address our blueprints. Naturally, different species will have a range of shapes according to seasons and locations. Polar bears put on huge reserves of fat to sustain them through hibernation, but by the time spring appears they are light enough to hunt their prey again. However, their extremes are within a set range. And those variations account for a very changeable habitat.

It is interesting to note that overweight wild animals are rarely seen. This is for three main reasons:

1. First of all, overweight animals are less able to run away from predators.

2. Secondly, underweight animals will be weak and unable to fight off their hunters.

3. Thirdly, and of most relevance to humans, their body blueprints have not been interfered with by concepts of fashion, and therefore remain unchanged. We are aware that domestic animals will become overweight when fed as if they are human.

The first two reasons are linked to survival, and that is the one fundamental purpose of life. We need to survive in our own generation and the next. For hundreds of thousands of years we have lived among our predators and prey. We have lived in a variety of lands and climates, and still do. Yet we are soft bodied, we lack horns, fangs, claws and scaly armour. How have we stayed alive as a species? The answer is that we are magnificent at surviving and our systems for keeping us alive are perfect.

Yet, tragically, we have an enemy that is all pervading and highly dangerous. It is called civilisation and it threatens us and our offspring. It even endangers our planet. Civilisation has stopped us from hunting for our food. It has tied us to telephones, televisions, desks and computer keyboards.

Before it became excessive, fat WAS good for us. Way back in time, in our cave-dwelling years, humans needed to store fat for the long winters and for when times would be hard. Men needed fat to sustain them during a long and unsuccessful hunting trip. Mothers needed stores of fat in order to survive and suckle their children. Children restricted the time available for mothers to search for food.

Above all, the need to survive famines was paramount. Fifty thousand years ago, life was hard and perilous. The body's ability to store fat is about survival, and we have been good at surviving as a species until our whole pattern of life was changed by imposed standards of attractiveness, fashion and chic. The natural systems that have kept us alive for hundreds of thousands of years seem to work against us in modern times. That is mostly because we work against them. We are a species that has lived, pretty much unchanged, for hundreds of thousands of years. The great thing is that we are still here. We have survived, and fat is part of that success.

The key to weight and shape control lies in the recognition of our successful animal roots. We are then able to accept an understanding of our blue-prints and our potential to change them. Throughout history fat has helped to keep us alive. It has acted as insulation. It has been an energy store. It has enabled us to endure famines. It has been our savings account for rainy days.

Money has the very much the same purpose that fat used to in that we save it and spend it to buy food. However, we have retained the need to store fat as well. We can never have too much money but we can have too much fat.

When we look back fifty thousand years to how we were when our unconscious minds and our bodies took responsibility for our well-being, then we can see some startling facts about modern approaches to weight and shape. As with all other mammals, we have the natural capability to fluctuate through the seasons of the year. Other animals acquire stores of fat before winter in order to survive hibernation. We had to do the same, but as we did not hibernate our reserves were regulated within our need to be mobile enough to scavenge during the lean months.

Imagine, for a moment, a woman sitting at the entrance to her cave fifty thousand years ago. Her shape was controlled more by her need to stay alive rather than by any thoughts of health or fashion. She probably gave very little conscious thought to her shape. She had no mirrors, scales or comprehension of her personal weight.

Only in more modern times would external ideals about shape arrive from fashion magazines, films, television and peer pressure. So, way back in time, our cave woman would have been content.

When winter arrived and food became short then she would have relied upon her body fat to remain alive, and if she had children, to keep them alive with her breast milk. She was unable to nip out to the local supermarket to top up her larder. Had the winter progressed for longer than usual then she would starve. A famine would have begun. If she survived, by the time that food became available again, she would have been very thin.

When food became more plentiful then she would have had the urge to eat to replace the fat she had lost. The crisis would have changed her blueprint to make her larger so that if another food shortage happened she would be better able to survive. Her fat store was now greater, or in modern terminology, she had become fatter.

Never assume that this only applied tens of thousands of years ago. This pattern applied until very recently. We can consider how similar they are to the life-styles in the 19th century for Europeans and for the American settlers. They even apply in the poorer countries of today. In the Western world, food only became very abundant a good few years after the Second World War.

It is this very survival system of storing fat that makes people put on weight after going on a diet. This is at the root of the classic 'yo-yo' dieting process. Our brains, our minds, cannot differentiate between a life threatening famine and the self-imposed diet. A diet is beyond the remit of the older parts of the brain. The effect of a diet is to evoke an unconscious feeling of danger, the famine response. The biological answer is to increase reserves of fat in order to ensure survival.

In those early days of human existence people lacked refrigerators or deep-freezers. They had no supermarkets down the valley. Everything our forebears ate had to be found from nature. The one safe place in which food would have been stored was in mother. She had the capacity to store food as fat that could be expressed back to the children as breast milk. It is likely that her children would have used her in the same way modern children use a vending machine!

Leonid Brezhnev (1906-1982), the ex-general secretary of the Soviet

Union is reported to have been breastfed by his mother to the age of 5 because he was a sickly child and times were hard. Even today there would be no choice for a mother in breast feeding her offspring or have them die from starvation.

Mothers seem to have an urge to finish leftover food from their children. Does this strike a chord with your client? The vast majority of mothers of young children seem to feel the drive to clear plates, or to cook a little extra when feeding their children. Way back in time there was nowhere to store food for the next day without risk of contamination except in mother. She could then give the stored fat back as milk. Never be revolted, it is a sign of our wonderful heritage.

When we look back at primeval life-styles, we can see why men and women store fat in different bodily locations. Men as the hunters of larger prey needed extra mobility to escape the other predators and to catch their own food. They would have stored fat on their fronts and backs. It is always strange to see how thin the legs of overweight men are when spotted on a beach.

Women would have been situated more around the homestead in order to guard their children. They would have foraged and hunted locally. Therefore women could store fat in a circle around their bodies from the chest to the thighs as they needed less mobility and were the source of milk for their infants.

Back in our old family, when the weather started to turn colder then the need to store food as fat would have become greater. The nights becoming longer and the subsequent gloominess made us turn to foods that contained sugars and fats. Call it general anxiety, or the need for greater security, but the drive to consume food grew. If we take the phrase 'comfort eating' and re-name it 'security eating', then the picture becomes clearer. It is the result of the knowledge that winter was drawing closer. They were the times when food became scarcer.

This is why people will lose weight and then regain it quickly after circumstances such as a separation, divorce, bereavement and so on. Fat reserves are then added in case it happens again. This relates to the loss of a hunter/gatherer and it stimulates the need to save fat to last out the future days of possible hardship.

Back in time, when we went out and found food growing on bushes or when we had killed an animal, we had two main urges. The first was to consume our bounty straight away because if we went back later then other animals would have eaten what had been left.

The second was to get out of there as quickly as possible before we became prey to the predators that were also hunting for food. So when we eat quickly we tend to consume more. The stomach is a very flexible thing that will expand to carry whatever is pushed into it.

When we eat slowly we put our minds back into the cave where there was little to eat or do. The moral of the story is to slow down when eating. This is the secret of Mediterranean diets where families will enjoy a long, slow main meal at lunchtime rather than rush through a big dinner in the evening.

The need to survive still exists. We worry about our work, our families, old age, our pensions, health-care, war, terrorism and just about everything. Our civilised ways have given us misgivings about life. In our modern lands of plenty, we store food as fat as if we had to exist for months on our own resources.

The major way in which your body shape is controlled is by metabolism. Some people will burn food at a higher rate than others in order to maintain their blueprint. Other people will burn food at a lower rate.

According to studies into appetite regulation, the daily intake of food is highly variable and correlates poorly with energy usage. Despite this, over long periods of time body weights are usually stable in most adults.

Going back fifty thousand years again, it would have been pointless to burn 1500 calories per day during a famine. Soon the reserves of fat would have been used and our cave dwellers would have died. It is much more likely that in order to hold onto body shape, or reserves of fat, metabolism would have slowed.

In modern times, when a person reduces their calorie intake during a diet, then the metabolism slows to maintain the blueprint shape as much as possible. This is called 'metabolic shift'. This is why dieters will become lethargic and miserable. Their metabolism has slowed to ensure the lowest possible usage of stored energy. The mind and body are screaming for the things that will replace the lost fat. The best thing to replace lost fat is fat! That is why dieters get cravings for certain products. They are, of course, sugar and fat. And then there is the ultimate mix of the two, chocolate.

We are different to steam trains! The energy from a certain amount of coal will fuel a boiler for the time to cover a certain distance. That is measurable. We are humans with a system that works to keep us alive. If we reduce our fuel intake then we will reduce the rate at which we burn it.

Reducing food intake only works when it is recognised by the mind and body as beneficial to survival. Therefore, when slow weight reduction at approximately seven pounds per month is translated as a movement towards a beneficial blueprint shape, it is accepted.

When weight loss is rapid it evokes the 'famine-response'. The system will be driven to add reserves of fat rather than to risk exposure to starvation.

The same applies to elimination diets. We are omnivores. We eat anything and everything. By doing so, we achieve a balance of nutrients, vitamins and minerals. When we eliminate certain food groups, we signal danger yet again. We are impelled to consume those things that our systems feel we are missing in order to sustain homeostasis.

We are not the only modern species that has become fatter. The animals that we farm are deliberately bred to be fattened so that there is more weight per lamb, pig, cow or chicken. This means that there is more fat to be consumed in meat in the twenty-first century than in the many thousands of years ago before farming became driven to produce 'bigger and fatter'.

A wild deer will be leaner because it has to compete for scarce food resources, and as mentioned earlier it would have been at a disadvantage if it were slow in escaping. As farming is an industry, the extra fat that is produced has to be disposed of in the food chain. Those excess fats are found in manufactured foods. It is found in pastries, pies, burgers, sausages and savoury snacks. Fats are used to cook foods such as French fries. Fat is added to our food in subtle ways. Not only do we have more food in our times, but we have a high proportion of fat in our diets.

The same point can be made about sugar. The sources of sweetness in our history were fruits and perhaps, more perilously, honey. Bees want to keep their external stores of sugars. Now we use sugar canes and beet to manufacture sugar which is used in our drinks, confections and as an additive to many foods. The high consumption of sugar is contributing to the huge increase in diabetes. The hypothalamus and pancreas have been over-burdened to the point where they are unable to cope.

So fats and sugars are a danger when consumed excessively. Yet fats and sugars are widely used and available. When they are eaten by overweight people they cause 'guilt-trips'. Those feelings of remorse add to anxiety. Anxiety leads to comfort/security eating. That leads to an increase of fat and sugar intake. That leads to weight gain. Weight gain leads to 'guilt-trips' and so on.

So people go on crash diets and count calories in an attempt to slim. The yo-yo dieting cycle kicks in. More weight, more guilt, more food and more fat. The vicious circle is complete. And when obesity and diabetes and heart disease enter onto the scene, the circle is very vicious indeed.

We are able to control our body shapes rather than provoking the responses that work against them. By working with our inherent systems, we can encourage weight loss in the medium to longer term.

Although this will seem like a new approach to weight control, it is hundreds of thousands of years old. Only since we started interfering with our natural systems through the use of dieting has the need to regain control of our internal weight and shape mechanisms become of paramount importance.

We are told that we have five senses, namely sight, hearing, touch, smell and taste. They are the ones with which we are familiar. They are for becoming aware of the world outside our bodies. They allow us to become acquainted with our environment.

We actually have more than those five. They are the inner senses. They are the ways in which our bodies experience and regulate themselves internally. For example, we have a sense of balance, kinaesthesia. This is the sense that tells you which way-up you are. It is the one that gives you a feeling of movement, direction and orientation when you are in an aircraft.

Then there is another sense that is used in re-setting your body-shape-blueprint. It is called proprioception, from proprius meaning 'one's own' and perception, which gives you information about where you are in space. It gives you an internal perspective.

Getting to know what proprioception is.

Please do these exercises with your clients. It is important that you become familiar with this sense of bodily feedback.

Ask the client to extend the first finger on their right hand, while they extend their arm to the side. They should then close their eyes and touch the end of their nose with their extended digit. This is the sense that is used as a preliminary drink-drive test by the American police. People lose it when drunk. It is a sense that is relevant to weight or shape control because it is the awareness of where parts of us are in relation to the rest of us. It is easily switched into.

Without moving or touching, the client should 'feel' the sole of the left foot. This will be felt as a low tingle. The client is sending slow nerve impulses to the sole of the foot. Signals are then sent back to tell the client that it is there. It is like using radar to detect something and then to pinpoint its location. Again, without the client moving they should feel where their right hip is: then where the left hip is. Then they should become aware of the space between them. This body checking is going on all the time, but at an unconscious level. However we can switch our conscious thought into it at will. Clients can feel their shape within their own mind. This sensory information is being fed into the hypothalamus.

Next the client uses proprioception to feel the fat on the back of their upper arm as it is. Then, with the mind, they should feel the shape of that part of that arm as it will be like when they have reached their target shape.

This is the insight to weight and shape control. Presume that the feedback goes into a mental processor, which checks against a blueprint and then changes the system to maintain a shape. This processor is the hypothalamus. Of course, we are unable to see an actual blueprint in a person's brain, but it can be seen within our mind's-eye or, for some people, felt with the mind's hand.

The good news is that we can consciously change our blueprints, and when that is done, bodies will change their shapes.

Blueprints are re-drawn with visualisation and proprioception. The client becomes aware of every part of their body bit by bit from the shape they are now to the shape that they would like to be, within reason.

Within reason is important because the mind and body work for survival. Remember that super-model shapes are for selling clothes, rather than for copying! If your client visualises and feels to be at an unhealthy body shape, then they run the risk of problems.

CHANGING THE BLUEPRINT

COMMENCEMENT DATE:
CURRENT WEIGHT:
TARGET WEIGHT:
DIFFERENCE:
TARGET DATE *:
TARGET DATE 'PICTURE' **
* Calculate the target date by dividing the weight difference by 7 pounds, or 3.2 kilos. This will give you the number of months in which your client should achieve the target shape when they follow the instructions given on the recording. Add these months, or part months, to the commencement date to give the target date.
** Now associate that date with a real point in time. For example, a birthday, anniversary, a holiday or a season. Perhaps something like the appearance of flowers in their garden. Do whatever you can to lock in their target date to an actual point of time.

1.   First of all, write down the client's current weight in a copy of the grid above
2.   Now write down the client's <u>realistic</u> target weight.
3.   Work out the difference in pounds or kilograms.
4.   Your client should aim to lose weight at the rate of 7 pounds, or 3.2 kilos per month. Remember that losing weight at a faster rate runs the risk of evoking the 'famine response'.

Along with the other suggestions that you will make there should be some about taking a small but progressively increasing amount of exercise. Exercise is important as it will consume energy but, more importantly, it distracts from client boredom, one reason why people snack and nibble, and it gives a better sense of well-being and therefore confidence to achieve.

Remember never use the 'not' word as you would create a negative suggestion. Part of your session will be suggestions about which foods to avoid where possible. Explain that rather than being taboo foods, the less quantity and the less frequently these foods are consumed, the easier losing weight will be.

Those foods should be those with fat and sugar in them, certainly those foods heavy with fat such as hard cheeses.

An important point is that you must maintain the client's feeling of security. When I do the weight control session I will use visualisation for the session. The proprioception part is on the CD that I give for the client to listen to on a weekly basis. This is because the idea of a client laying back with their eyes closed and in hypnosis imagining that they are feeling themselves all over seems to be totally inappropriate. This they do at home with the CD. In my office they should feel safe.

Those who want, and need, to lose substantially more and who are obese.
Obesity is a contemporary ailment. The reasons for obesity are many.

People who have been abused may put on weight for protection. Excess fat can also be seen as a repellent of sexual advances.

Bully victims want to be 'bigger' to avoid physical hurt. We are unable to make ourselves taller, but we can make ourselves wider. Fat may be perceived as armour against punches.

Please note: There is no suggestion whatsoever that all obese people have been abused sexually or physically.

Size, as in the build and height of a person, is almost certainly to do with genetics and nurture. However, the amount of fat that is carried by a person is probably more to do with other influences. Overweight people blame genetics as a 'get-out' clause. If a person's parents are overweight, they can blame their ill-fortune on their ancestors and they will be less mentally able to tackle their own size problems.

It might be worth considering that in our survival make-up we might have a predisposition to copy the shapes of those people around us. If they are carrying a lot of fat, then perhaps it indicates that they live in a high risk valley, in primeval terms. Therefore it would seem to make sense that we imitate their shapes to further our own chances of continued existence.

We have already established that anxiety relates to eating habits such as bingeing and comfort eating. The famine response may be evoked when times seem stressful. Bingeing and comfort eating occur when people feel that hard times are happening, or are coming. Bingeing is similar to primeval feasting. Feasting is a feature within our history. Perhaps finishing food before it went bad, perhaps sharing the outcome of a hunt. They were all to add fat to the personal store in anticipation of 'leaner' days. We still do it in mid-winter to this day, but we call it Christmas or something else.

When clients are dramatically overweight the first avenue to explore is the reason why. Analysis is necessary to explore history and to find a cause. If a client presents with a major weight issue there is something that motivated him/her to see you. They will be fairly open when talking about their experiences so your job is to work with them to find resolution.

This will take a number of sessions and you can arrange to meet on a monthly basis to review the weight loss. This gives an incentive to the client to keep on losing weight at a gentle rate after the initial cause has been explored.

Those who have been told to lose weight by somebody in authority such as a dance instructor.
This is sadly annoying. When a client who is very thin rather than anorexic arrives to see you because they MUST lose weight as told by a

dance instructor or by a theatrical agent, please avoid screaming with anger because you will frighten the client!

How you deal with this is a fragile thing. On one hand you can destroy a career if you refuse and on the other you can potentially destroy a life.

You have little right to question the instructor or agent who would refuse to talk to you anyway. You can only help the client by suggesting that he/she seeks an alternative instructor.

The client should really talk to a doctor who would have more chance of making the instructor or agent see sense, sadly.

Those who want to lose weight because they have an eating disorder.
At the other extreme, the refusal to grow can be an attempt to cling onto childhood, those 'safer' times. This has a bearing on the low-weight problems associated with anorexia and bulimia. Anorexics are hard nuts to crack. They seem to carry a cocktail of problems and cause. Some range from almost a body dysmorphic problem where they are searching for bodily perfection and they perceive themselves to be fat, grotesque and ugly. Some have been abused and want to punish the body.

Without copping out, this is an area where specialist help is required and training beyond reading a book is essential. **Eating disorders can, and do, kill.**

STRICTLY FOR THERAPISTS

PART FIVE

Techniques for:

Breathing
Language
Posture

The following techniques have been added from The Secret Language of Hypnotherapy. My choice was to either add them, but rewritten for therapists, or to omit them as they have been published before.

I consider them to be so very important for the effective treatment of clients that they had to be included even if you have read them before in my other book.

Breathing

When the breath wanders the mind also is unsteady. But when the breath is calmed the mind too will be still, and the yogi achieves long life. Therefore, one should learn to control the breath.
~Svatmarama, *Hatha Yoga Pradipika*

Teaching your clients to breathe correctly is very important. In this way you give them a way to relax and a way to cope.

In history, breathing was considered to be such an important part of life that the word 'spirit' comes from 'spiritus', the Latin word for breathe, as in respiration. It is also the root word for inspiration. However, it is one of the things that is often overlooked, or misunderstood. The effect of the breath is at the very heart of problems and, happily, solutions.

Breathing in the correct way has been taught for centuries. To the Yogis of India the word 'prana' means the element to which all other substances might finally be reduced as is the spirit of life in Western culture. Regulation of the breath is known as 'pranayama' and it is practised for mental and physical wellbeing.

In China, the same thing is known as 'Chi', as in Tai Chi, a routine of slow meditative physical exercise for relaxation and balance and health. In other words, the practice and benefits of breathing correctly have been known for thousands of years for spiritual (mental) and bodily well-being. However, modern culture has dictated that we should have body shapes that emphasise the chest and minimize the stomach. That is the very shape that inhibits correct breathing.

We breathe from the moment that we are born so we feel that we know how to do it correctly. And we do. After all, we are alive! As a point of interest, when we die, we expire! I get looks of surprise when I talk to clients about the correct ways to breathe.

197

The lungs are misunderstood! We tend to think of them as a pair of balloon-like bags in our chests that take oxygen in and push carbon dioxide out. They are, in fact, complex excretory organs. They are made from tubes and cavities that allow the exchange of gases. They remove many waste products as well as carbon dioxide, which is why we can smell garlic on people's breath. The little cavities, called alveoli, work constantly and are independent of the respiratory, or breathing, cycle. The process of gas exchange is dependent upon their concentrations. Waste gases either remain in the lungs until flushed out by breathing or are re-absorbed into the bloodstream when the concentration increases. The re-absorption of those exhaust gases can make people feel anxious, uncomfortable, nervous and irritable. The breathing rate is controlled by blood acidity levels so an increase in carbon dioxide in the blood stream increases carbonic acid levels. This, in turn, increases the rate at which we breathe to eliminate excesses of carbon dioxide to achieve a natural balance. However, hyperventilation occurs when carbon dioxide, and carbonic acid, levels fall too low which constricts the blood vessels restricting its flow to the brain.

Sufferers from panic attacks are often told to take deep breaths to prevent hyperventilation. However, the instructions about how to do this are often very often counter-productive. Some experts appear to misunderstand what they instructing their clients or patients to do!

We are taught from an early age that neatness is important in body posture. If you ask your client take a deep breath, as they were instructed by their parents, schoolteachers and others whose intentions are to produce that neatness, then they will probably breathe into the high chest. This produces tension and stiffness in the neck and shoulder muscles, and a drawing in of the stomach.

If you simulate the position that you would adopt under attack, it is the same. The neck and shoulders tighten to protect the throat and the back of the head. The stomach muscles tighten to protect the soft organs of the abdomen, the liver, kidneys and spleen from injury. The legs cross to protect the genitals.

In this way, poor advice to breathe deeply actually imitates the posture of somebody under threat. Remember that panic, anxiety, stress and anger are responses to a threat, whether real or imaginary. It is important to teach your clients to breathe deeply into the abdomen rather than the high chest. In this way your clients will signal to their minds that they are safe, and thereby evoke a recovery response that counters those feelings of anxiety. Breathing involves two sets of muscles.

The intercostal muscles.
These extend downwards and connect the ribs. When they are contracted the ribs are pulled upwards and outwards to enlarge the rib cage (thoracic cavity). These are the breathing muscles that predominate during the anxiety state when the blood needs to be well oxygenated. They can work rapidly to produce panting which can lead to hyperventilation where the blood is over oxygenated and leads to tingling in the extremities of the body and light-headedness. This accounts for the high number of panic attack victims who are admitted to the cardio-vascular units of hospitals.

The diaphragm.
This is a dome shaped muscle at the base of the lungs. When contracted it 'flattens' and causes air to flow into the lungs. Its effect is to enlarge the thoracic cavity in length. The diaphragm is the muscle that sucks air into the lower parts of the lungs and in turn, it flushes out waste gases that collect there. This type of breathing is indicative of a relaxed state. It is the natural way to breathe. Every child breathed in this way until school age.

Breathing, theoretically, includes the use of both sets of muscles to ensure an entrance of fresh air and the expulsion of waste products throughout the lungs. The high-chest breathing which occurs during anxiety states involves the use of the intercostal muscles and the locking of the diaphragm as a result of taught stomach muscles.

The exercises that follow will encourage your clients to use their diaphragms as the main muscle for respiration.

4 x 4 BREATHING

STARTING POSITION Get your client to lie on their back on the floor. They should be reassured that they are safe to do so. Make sure they are decently dressed. Hand them a medium sized book to put over the stomach just at the point where the rib cage ends. NEVER place it on the client yourself. Ensure that their neck and shoulder muscles are loose and relaxed. The client should relax their stomach muscles.	**START**
STEP ONE Ask the client to breathe deeply into their stomach to raise the book as if they were trying to lift it to touch the ceiling for the duration of your slow count of four. Ask the client to keep their chest as still as possible.	**LIFT** 1...2...3...4 **(Please note: Whilst breathing in avoid inflating the upper parts of your lungs because they will fill automatically.)**
STEP TWO The client should hold the book, in the raised position, for your slow count of four of the same duration as in step one.	**HOLD** 1...2...3...4
STEP THREE The client then breathes out to lower the book for the same count of four. Get them to imagine that they are lowering it to touch their backbones.	**DOWN** 1...2...3...4
STEP FOUR The client then leaves their lungs feeling 'empty' for a count of four.	**LEAVE ON BACKBONE** 1...2...3...4

As we are conditioned to breathe with the high chest, concentrating on using the diaphragm will result in a balanced breathing practice. The above, the 4 x 4 Breathing Method, is a superb exercise to teach your clients. Ensure that the client is safe and **NEVER** touch them or place the book on their stomachs. They must do that for themselves.

The counting for the client should be done by the therapist for two cycles and then the clients are asked to do it for two cycles themselves with their eyes closed.

ASK YOUR CLIENT IF THEY HAVE MEDICAL PROBLEMS BEFORE DOING THE EXERCISES. IF THEY HAVE, THEY SHOULD CONSULT THEIR DOCTOR. THIS REFERS TO THE BACK, KNEES AND JOINTS AS WELL AS THE LUNGS.

There are three benefits that should be explained to the client:

1 The fight or flight response is caused by a part of the mind that is beyond conscious control. There is an opposing system also beyond conscious control that can be tricked into operation. Because the client is lying on the floor they are feeling slightly vulnerable. This vulnerability in a controlled situation is reminiscent of the cave dweller being in a safe place after being chased by a predator. The body needed to come down to a state where energy consumption was low and where repairs could take place. When relaxed the immune system is maximised. The position they are in replicates those circumstances and the relaxation response (the parasympathetic branch of the autonomic nervous system) kicks in.

2 The exercise strengthens the diaphragm. This is a big muscle that weakens when underused. When it flattens out it also massages the gut from above, aiding digestion. This means that, with the increased levels of relaxation, this has a double benefit for sufferers from IBS.

3 Whilst concentrating on breathing in a fairly unusual way, the client's mind will be distracted from the worries that caused them to be tense.

201

As a species we are vulnerable at four points on the body. They are the back of the neck, the throat, the soft abdominal organs (liver, kidneys, spleen etc.) and our genitals. The above exercise exposes them. (A horribly ambiguous word that, in this case, means in a covered and decent way.)

CATS AND DOGS

Ask your clients to observe their pets. They know how to breathe because they do it naturally without regard to the fashionable appearance of their bodies. When relaxed and safe they use the diaphragm to breathe. When they are running you will notice rapid, high-chest breathing. If they say "walkies" to their sleeping dogs, which is heard in dog language as 'let's go hunting', the diaphragmatic breathing will immediately change to panting. The dog is increasing the oxygen in its bloodstream to ready it for action.

Every animal on this planet breathes correctly apart from the human who lives in our modern culture. The desire for big chests and flat stomachs has caused modern society to adopt the breathing patterns that promote anxiety and stress disorders.

EXASPERATION!

When we are irritated by something, we often take a deep breath in, hold it and then breathe out with a sigh of exasperation. This is a natural phenomenon that, in our primeval days, took us from a high-energy state to a recovery state in brief moments. We can use this response without being irritated. It is similar in effect to the 'explosive relaxation' technique described later, but with a focus on breathing rather than posture.

OPERA SINGERS AND SWIMMERS

An opera singer has to be able to sing long complicated word structures as well as high, low and long notes.

Like a swimmer, the opera singer has to master breathing. Whereas it is difficult to imitate the swimmer's breathing patterns, it is easier to play a charade as an opera singer!

Encourage your clients to take deep breaths and pretend to sing long notes. This should be done in private rather than in your office! This helps them to automatically use both the intercostal and diaphragmatic muscles.

In TV talent shows the singing coaches will concentrate on diaphragmatic breathing, I am sure. This helps the singer to sing AND to relax in what could be one of the most stress causing scenarios that we can imagine.

Language

It's a strange world of language in which skating on thin ice can get you into hot water. ~Franklin P. Jones

When we are thinking, it is like having a conversation within our own minds. This is our internal dialogue. Those thoughts are 'flavoured' by our emotions. We run a process of risk evaluation at the same time. When we are walking we recognise ruts in the road, or dark corners where dangers might lurk. However, when we worry, we think about problems that might become reality without having rational justification.

We know that thoughts can change feelings. Fear is an emotion. Those fears that seem to come from nowhere have their origins in unconscious thoughts rather than from a recognised stimulus. Clients react as if the threat were a real thing. Rather than thoughts they become 'feelings'. Yet when those thoughts are of pleasure, we all relax.

The language that clients use for their internal and external dialogue is important for their well-being and for dealing with the problems that underlie their anxiety. Within modern culture there are four things relating to language which work against us, but which we can use to our advantage when we know the secrets.

1. We live in a society that sells problems for a living.

Can you imagine taking your car to a showroom where you are told that the vehicle you have is perfect? No!

They might suggest that the mileage is high, or the engine size is unsuitable, or that the fuel consumption is uneconomical. They will identify and explain the 'problems' that you have and then they will solve them by selling you a new car. This applies to most trades.

Even salaries are paid because if a position were vacant, the company would have a problem in getting its necessary work done. We survive by solving problems.

2. We use words too cheaply.

We sustain our personal problems by the poor use of language. That is, we use words too cheaply. We pepper our speech with brief idioms that communicate on a superficial level, but have different deep-seated meanings. My favourite example of poor language that is counter-productive came from a client who said: "Perhaps I really ought to try to think more positively!" That sentence contained all the reasons why she would find it difficult to do so.

The words 'perhaps', 'I really', 'ought' and 'try' are weak rather than positive. They are 'failure' words. They appear to state a positive objective but they infer that the goal will be missed. If the intention is firm then the sentence becomes, "I think positively."

3. We like negatives!

We tend to use strange constructions that are based on double negation. Why do we say, "that's not a bad idea" rather than "that's a good idea", for example?

Negatives are necessary for rational disciplines. Mathematics has to have the concept of negatives to work, but we are dealing with emotions. As you will see later, negatives are unable to dismiss problems but they potentially intensify them.

4. We make our lives conditional.

We make statements to ourselves and then accept them as solid truths. Superstitions are a good example. "If I walk under a ladder then I will be unlucky" or "a black cat crossing my path is a good omen" or a bad one in some cultures! We make our lives conditional. If X happens then Y will follow.

This happens with anxiety states. "If I go to the supermarket then I will have a panic attack." I have even heard the statement, "I know that I will get a panic attack two and a half hours after taking my beta-blocker." Surprise, surprise! She did until we changed her language. Suggestions are quickly made and adhered to. When we make the wrong choices with suggestions then we pay a high price.

BREAKING OUT OF THINKING TRAPS

Self-talk is full of traps. Most people have heard of the word 'affirmation', a positive phrase or suggestion aimed at changing the ways in which we think about ourselves. The most famous one is "Everyday, in every way, I am getting better and better." However, very few people actually use positive affirmations. Most of us are very adept at using negative ones by accident! We develop and hold onto erroneous beliefs that distort and change our behaviours and attitudes.

Sadly, clients are wonderful in reinforcing negatives by their thinking. When they make negative suggestions to themselves then they run a huge risk of believing them. Things like the following need to be ruthlessly destroyed:
'I am unlucky.'
'I am ugly.'
'I am a loser.'
'I will get fired because I am useless at my job.'

There is a way to break the negativity of your client's self-talk. We get them to use very positive techniques for changing their language, which in turn modifies their thinking, emotions and reactions. These are based on eliminating negative words and conditions. We encourage clients to replace them with a language and thinking that contains beneficial intention.

The rules and steps are simple and easy to remember.

Look at the sentence 'I will NOT panic (or get angry/become anxious/get stressed, etc.) in the supermarket' (or in the car, at the restaurant, at work, on a date, etc.) This seems as if it will work.

However, within that short sentence there are three fundamental errors of thought that will bring about the opposite response. From working through this example, we see how to turn client goals into language that communicates the correct message to their minds.

1. 'I WILL' puts the hoped for solution into the future. The future is tomorrow, next week, next year, whatever. This tells us that whereas relief will be found, it is unlikely that it will help them <u>now</u>. Putting that hope into the future reinforces the problem that they currently have.

So the first rule and step is to place their problem into the past tense.

If it WAS a problem, then it follows that it has gone. Their mind gives them the unconscious positive suggestion, or affirmation, that they need. Then they put the solution into the present tense by using the words 'I' and 'NOW'.

The affirmation then becomes: 'I used to panic in the supermarket (or whatever) but NOW, I feel calm, confident and in control.'

If the client finds that their mind tells them that their problem still exists, then persuade the client to argue with it! They must repeat their affirmation over and over.

2. The second rule is to lose the small word 'NOT'. This includes you, the therapist when making suggestions. Although we know what positive suggestions are, we fail to use them. Instead, anxiety sufferers use negative suggestions accidentally. These maintain the problem rather than giving them a solution. When we are thinking about behaviours, our minds seem to be unable to recognise negatives. When we use the word 'NOT' we often create the opposite outcome to that which is desired. Let me give an example: 'Do NOT think of blue elephants!'

It is likely that you thought of blue elephants. It therefore follows that the sentence 'I will NOT panic in the supermarket' is understood as 'I WILL panic in the supermarket' because the instruction is contained after the word 'NOT' in the words 'panic in the supermarket'. The word 'not' has no effect in changing that instruction. The blue elephant example told you, after the word 'NOT', to think of blue elephants.

So, use a sentence that affirms what the client wants to happen rather than using a negative in an attempt to negate the unwanted effect. To repeat, lose the word 'NOT' from your and your clients' thoughts. In its place, state the result that you and they want in positive terms.

A quick note. Whereas the word 'not' is to be avoided in suggestions and self talk dialogue, it is permitted in negating things as in 'blue is not green' and in descriptions. It is to be avoided in suggestions.

3. The third rule, and next step, is get the client to omit any reference to the problem when they are used to referring to it the past tense and when they have stopped using the word 'not'. The last part of the sentence is a reminder of the problem and it is emphasised. '...panic in the supermarket.' It tells them to do what they want to avoid. Never feed a problem by talking or thinking about it. Starve it to death. Make it an exile, something that used to cause upsets but which has now been eliminated. Remove the problem and encourage the clients to tell themselves what they want to happen. 'In the supermarket (or in the car, at the restaurant, at work, on a date, etc.), I am calm, confident and in control.

PUTTING IT ALL TOGETHER:

1. Make suggestions positive, current and relevant to the solution. Ignore the problem completely. It is something that the client used to have, but now they are fine.

2. Avoid certain other words such as 'perhaps', 'ought', 'should', 'maybe', 'if', 'might', 'probably' and 'try'. These imply either failure or weakness.

3. Make internal dialogue strong and assertive. The clients tell themselves what they want to be by telling themselves that what they wanted to be in the future is how they actually are, now.

Words to avoid in your suggestions and in your clients' thinking:
• Try. Implies failure. Remember that when somebody says that they will try to see you at 3 o'clock, that gives you at least ten more minutes before they will actually arrive.
• Not. Creates a negative suggestion as already mentioned.
• But. When used in the present tense to explain why something will fail. In this way, 'but' creates the negative reinforcement of the problem. For example "I would like to drive on motorways, but I panic."
• Perhaps. Conditional expectation of failure as in "perhaps I will get better".
• Might. Conditional expectation of failure.
• Maybe. Conditional expectation of failure.
• Should. Conditional expectation of failure.

Words to use cautiously
• All words which put action or intent into the future. They maintain the problem in the present time. However, if they reflect an intent that was previously missing and a time frame, they are useful. For example "I will go to the doctor tomorrow" or "I can relax when I visit the hairdresser in an hour's time."
• Can. A positive word that refers to the future but is sometimes conditional.
• Will. A positive word that refers to the future.
• If. This makes the intent conditional. An example of bad usage is, "if I meet somebody new, then I will be anxious." An example of better usage is, "if I use positive language then I will be in control." However, it is best to say, "I use positive language and I am in control, now." (See below.)

Words to use:
• (I) Do. A positive word in the present time.
• (I) Am. A positive word in the present time.

- Now. A positive word in the present time.
- But (when following placing the problem into the past tense.) Used this way, 'but' creates a positive affirmation. For example "I used to worry about driving on motorways, but now I feel calm, confident and in control."
- Avoid. This is a word of positive intent. "I used to get angry with myself, but now I avoid criticising myself by recognising my true value."
- As. A conditional word that implies a result. For example, as you read this book you find it is helping you to improve your proficiency.

ENCOURAGE CLIENTS TO:
1. Place problems into the past tense and the positive outcomes into the 'here-and-now'.
2. Lose the word 'not', and any other 'weak' words.
3. Then, omit any reference to the problem. Define the solution in 'strong' words.

WHEN THEY CHANGE THE LANGUAGE OF THOUGHTS, THEN;
Minds becomes more relaxed;
Then body postures change;
Then breathing changes;
Then life changes...for the better.

Posture

**Health is a state of complete harmony of the body, mind and spirit.
When one is free from physical disabilities and mental distractions,
the gates of the soul open. B.K.S. Iyengar**

When we feel fearful or aggressive, our bodies tighten. Just as there is
communication between our minds and our bodies, there is interaction
between our body positions and our emotions. When we adopt certain
positions we tell our minds that there is a potential 'alert state', and our
mental processes react accordingly. This is fairly obvious when it
involves negative effects, but the body/mind relationship can be used
in a positive way in order to mediate the fight or flight response.

We are very similar to chimpanzees, gorillas and orang-utans, yet
none of them stand to attention or sit up straight, apart from us
humans. Only we have to eat with our elbows off the table!

Our body postures relate to our feelings of well-being. There are two
phrases, which exemplify this connection between body attitude and
state of mind, 'up-tight' and 'laid-back'.

When we are tense, nervous or anxious our bodies tighten up. This is
because we are in the early stages of the fight or flight response. We
feel under threat from something that is outside ourselves or from that
feeling of dread that can grow from our minds. The closing up of our
bodies protects us, to some extent, when under physical threat.

To feel how our muscles are linked when under attack, do the
following. Relax your neck, shoulder and stomach muscles. Now
tighten your stomach muscles. Notice how your neck and shoulders
tighten in sympathy. You can do it the other way around. There is no
direct connection between the muscles, but the signals from one part of
your body are transmitted through your mind to the other.

The same thing happens when you extend an arm and make a tight fist. The tension is felt all the way up to the neck.

When our bodies tense, our minds read the signs and start to worry about what the assumed threat might be. Think about the body positions of anxiety sufferers even when they are in a safe place. Likewise, the client who has been bullied will sink the head into the shoulders. The stomach muscles are firmed. The legs and arms are crossed. All without reason. We could understand the body posture if the victim were surrounded by thugs, but even when secure, the body reflects the possibility of being attacked. We can use the body to persuade the mind that there is no need to panic, that the best response is to relax and recover, to be 'laid-back'.

The significance of an awareness of body position and muscle tone in controlling anxiety is that when the body feels prepared for its assumed attack then the mind is involved and sets the fight or flight response into motion. Tension in the body promotes tension in the mind.

The contrary applies, however. When the body is relaxed, it signals to the mind that it is safe and the recovery response kicks in. We can consciously control the positions and tension of our muscles; therefore we actually have conscious control of the recovery response, albeit in an indirect way. We trick the system that is supposed to be beyond conscious control into action.

As written earlier, we are no more than primeval animals in modern dress. We still live in the pattern of our ancient ancestors. There are situations in our lives that remind us, at some level, of our earlier days and we respond accordingly.

In a society where food is fairly abundant it is difficult to imagine how we must have been when dividing the spoils of a hunt. Yet we watch hyenas and lions snarling at, and biting each other in wildlife documentaries on TV. We see animals fighting off rivals in the mating process. We were like that, so it will come as no surprise that we become tense and anxious in social situations that involve food and courtship.

I have seen many clients who were distressed when eating in restaurants, or who were unable to swallow their meals. This unconscious worry about the possible aggression of others can lie at the heart of the panicking supermarket shopper where we 'take' self-service food, which we feel others want. It is different in a small store where we are served. Our ancestors would have felt comfortable when handed food, without risk, by the elders after they had first taken their fill.

We observe the bullying which takes place in schools as children play domination and submission roles. We see the worries that some people have in crowds where others are seen as unfriendly and frightening. The work situation is often difficult to cope with when colleagues and bosses are reflecting early social hostilities. Stress is more often caused by people in the workplace rather than by the work itself.

When we feel threats that are real or implied, then we close our bodies to protect our existence. Our muscles tighten and our minds race. This is the fight-or-flight response in action. Release the tension, open your body and signal your mind to calm down. When you do this, you relax because you stimulate the recovery response into action.

It is useful to watch pets when they are resting. They will sleep in a very exposed position when feeling safe and secure. Children, before being told how to sit like adults, will relax on the floor in front of the television. This is our natural and instinctive positioning until we are made to change to conform to adult standards of order. So copy children and pets. Learn from them. Lounge around and be casual. Then you will feel more relaxed. Show your clients to be calm and comfortable, or 'laid-back'.

EXPLOSIVE RELAXATION

This exercise teaches your clients to recognise that instant relief is possible when they are feeling tense. Get them to take up a tight position and suddenly explode into the exposed position shown in the 'BE LAID-BACK' frame below. All tension disperses instantly and they receive a sense of peace. They can enhance this feeling with slow and deep abdominal breathing, described in the breathing section.

Here is how you do it:
Ask the client to sit on an armchair or comfortable couch. Make sure it is sturdy enough to take their body weight when they flop backwards.

They tighten their muscles to adopt a rigid body position. They place the hands together palm to palm. Then they pull their feet back, close to the chair. They close their eyes and adopt the 'up-tight' position.

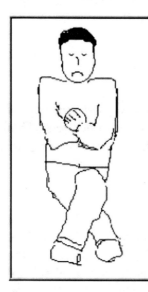

UP-TIGHT
This body position represents hiding from the environment, which includes people as well as animals and physical objects. We focus our vision into a stare (or close our eyes), tighten our muscles and protect ourselves.

When we sit in this 'up-tight' position our mind fears an attack and we become predisposed to anxiety or panic. The fear of anxiety or panic makes us even more tense, and so on.

They take a deep breath into their stomachs and hold it.

When you instruct them you count from 3 down to 1, and say, out loud, the word "NOW."

As you say this word, they should sprawl out. Their head goes back to the chair or couch. Their legs part in front of them by 18 inches or so as they make contact with the floor with their heels. Their arms fly out to the side, palms upwards.

As they relax there they can breathe gently through the navel. They are now 'laid-back'.

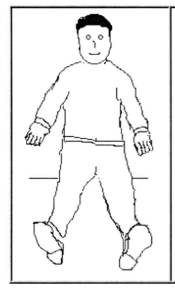

BE LAID-BACK

The clients 'expose' themselves to the environment. This opens up the paths for relaxed, diaphragmatic breathing.

This signals to their mind that their bodies are safe from threat. Their minds will perceive this and bring the recovery response into play which allows them to relax even more.

This is the positive feedback that their minds and bodies need in order to find relief from panic, anxiety, stress and anger.

You may have recognised that this position is very similar to that adopted by practitioners of meditation, the difference being that the calves of your client's legs are stretched outwards rather than the legs being bent at the knees in the lotus position. You will have taught your clients how to relax in a similar way to the way the Beatles did in India, but in a shorter space of time.

ENSURE THAT ANXIOUS AND PANICKY CLIENTS AVOID THE FOLLOWING:

1. Ankle crossing.
When at work, commuting or eating in restaurants, watch other people. The vast majority will have their legs crossed at the ankles with their feet tucked back below their knees. This is a sign of tension. It causes the leg muscles to tense and this is fed back to their minds. Clients should uncross their ankles and extend their feet forwards onto their heels. They should breathe using their diaphragms.

2. Badly set-up computer keyboards.

If your client uses a keyboard or laptop, review the position that they adopt when typing. Very often, screen angles will cause the neck to bend backwards which duplicates the 'under threat' position. Some people in open plan offices feel vulnerable when they have their backs to their colleagues. They should change orientation if this is a problem.

3. Dehydration.

Dehydration, such as that which follows drinking alcohol or large quantities of coffee, makes people feel anxious. Many people report having their first anxiety attack after drinking alcohol heavily during the previous evening. The solution for them is to avoid excess alcohol, to reduce coffee intake and/or to drink plenty of water.

4. Feeling trapped.

Feelings of being trapped are felt in a variety of situations including crowds, restaurants, cinemas, theatres, supermarkets, trains, aircraft and when driving. Techniques for changing language, posture and breathing practices are key factors in controlling the fight or flight response that follows exposure to the situation or feared object. Encourage clients to know and to believe that they are in control.

5. Food competition.

This has a primeval connection. Food has been such an important factor of life since history began that we become competitive in any situation where there is social interaction involving food. This includes restaurants and self-service stores and supermarkets. Even the check-out, the place where some people feel like rushing away, is the point which represents losing the product of the hunt to scavengers. In these situations, clients should remember that they are free of dissension over foodstuffs. There is plenty to go around. So much, in fact, that what we see on our plates or in our trolleys is always non-contentious, so they are safe.

6. Gripping.

There are specific situations where gripping an object can make people feel anxious. The tension of a vice-like grip tightens the muscles in the neck and shoulders. Then the stomach tenses and the body goes into an amber alert. From there, anything can happen! The common scenarios are the following:

- The steering wheel.

When driving, the client should hold the steering wheel gently as if holding the wrists of a baby. They must maintain control, obviously, but without clenching.

- The pram handle.

Again, the client can maintain control, but with a looser grip.

- The supermarket trolley handle.

If the client's load is heavy, a supermarket trolley can become difficult to control, so they must either shop more frequently, although this can become a nuisance and adds to anxiety, or, better still, they can ask their partner to push the trolley! Just loosening the grip helps.

- The golf club.

Gripping too tightly can cause enough tension to upset the swings of golfers. Another result is something called 'the yips', the inability to hit a putt on the green. If these are problems for sporting clients they should loosen the grip, breathe with the diaphragm, and above all, just enjoy a game that is supposed to be a pleasure.

7. Holding a newspaper in the air.
As with a steering wheel, holding a newspaper can tighten the neck and shoulders, bringing about a feeling of anxiety. Look at the stressed faces of commuting business people. When they get to their offices, they are feeling either timid or aggressive.

8. Hunching.
Anxious people hunch in many different situations. These include meeting others socially, being interviewed, sitting in restaurants, driving, working and sitting at home. They can be shown that they can stand or sit without tightening the neck, shoulders and stomach. As well as looking more relaxed, they will feel it.

9. Sexual/Social competition.
This is another point of primeval worry. Anxiety, jealousy and anger come from the fear that we might be attacked or have our mate stolen

from us. This is most easily seen in places where teenagers and singles meet. In these situations it is better to be with friends who offer security of numbers or to avoid places which have a reputation for trouble.

For mothers on a school run there is sometimes a worry about how others will regard their competence as mothers. They must learn that their child is the best in the world and that they are the person who raised him/her. Therefore your client is the best mum, ever.

10. **Wearing a collar and tie too tightly.**
Fashion works against us society. The brain needs a large amount of blood flowing through it. If we wear ties too tightly, or if collars are too small for our necks, then neckwear becomes a garrotte rather than clothing. A tight collar will also put pressure on the neck muscles so that clients tighten them to counteract the noose. This encourages neck and shoulder muscles to contract which, as we know, stimulates anxiety.

Where possible, anxious people should leave their ties off, or loosen them. This might go against the grain for an anxious person but with a looser collar they should become less anxious and they should also look at our business leaders like Richard Branson and successful men such as Simon Cowell. They rarely, if ever, wear ties.

PART SIX

Helpful Tips

Helpful Tips

Hand rising to face as an unconscious signal that a suggestion has been accepted.
A client's mind has to, sometimes, be convinced that a resolution has been accomplished. A method that I use is to relax the client and then do the following:

I ask the client's mind to allow me to ask it to change. Then I go through a routine where I talk to the 'unconscious part' of the mind. I ask it to change because the behaviour that is being carried out, i.e. panicking in certain situations is no longer protecting the client. I explain that the better course of action is to allow the client to relax on those occasions. Then I ask that part of the mind to make a signal to the client, and to me, that the change has taken place. The signal I ask for is for one of the hands, with no conscious effort, to gently rise to the face, touch it, and then return to where it was resting. I then say that this might take ten seconds, twenty seconds or longer and that all I want the client to consciously think about is whether it will be the left hand or right hand that makes the signal. I then say that I will be quiet for a while and wait for the signal.

If the client's hand rises I then ask the client to open their eyes and I will make small talk for a while. What I am looking for is for a hand to go to the face. When it does I will say, 'that was the signal.' I will say that the first had raise was a conscious desire for the mind to accept the change and that the real signal was made after they opened their eyes. I hand over a piece of paper that has the following written on it. 'The signal occurs after the eyes are opened when all conscious attention is taken away. It is like rubbing the nose, eye or mouth, usually unknowingly.'

The effect is amazing. The client will be surprised and will accept the suggestions hidden in the instructions. If, in the first stage, the hand stays still for more than a minute I will ask the client to open the eyes and I will wait for the real signal. This can be called ideo-motor signalling or whatever you like. The effect is powerful and effective in getting a client to accept that fundamental change has taken place.

Invisible watch induction
I do this as something to unblock resistance to hypnosis. If people ask where my watch is, in a sarcastic way, I will ask them to stare at my 'invisible' watch.

I describe it my using my hands. Then holding the chain in one hand I start the watch swinging from side to side while they look at it. I will ask if it is gold or silver and which colour the dial is. After a while I take my hands away and ask them to keep looking at the watch as it swings. Sooner or later eye fatigue creeps in and I make the suggestion that the eyelids are becoming heavier and will soon close and stay closed while the person slips into hypnosis. This works!

Then I will ask them to wake up and I will start a serious session. What has happened is that the person feels that I have been able to do something by using their imagination and the cynicism goes away. This, I must admit, is something that I only do on very rare occasions, maybe when a client arrives for an appointment, made by his wife, for me to 'make' him stop smoking. He wants to be able to go home and explain that his mind is too powerful to be influenced by a hypnotist!

Eyes and/or hands stuck. Trying leads to failure.
This is good for explaining the negative value of the word 'try'. It takes a leaf from the stage hypnotist's book, but I will tell the client that it has nothing to do with hypnosis.

Ask the client to hold their hands together, fingers interlocked and then turn them above their heads, palms skywards. Tell them you are going to tell them to **try** to separate their hands but they will be stuck together. Keep telling them to **try** and that their hands will be stuck together. After a while ask them to relax, and that they should return their hands to their starting position.

Before you do the next one, ensure that the client has no eye problems and they have no contact lenses in place.
Tell the client that, in a moment, you will put imaginary super-glue on their eyelids and when they close their eyes tightly the lids will be stuck together. Tell them that to avoid getting glue on their eyeballs they must keep staring at an imaginary TV screen on the inside of their forehead. When they have closed their eyes and rolled their eyeballs up tell them to keep staring at the screen and to try to open their eyes. They will be unable to do so.

Explain that both effects are based on physiology and language. The physiology is that the knuckles of the fingers make it difficult to part the hands and that the same blocks of muscles control the eyelids and the eyeballs. When the eyes are rolled up it is impossible to open closed eyes.

The purpose of this is to demonstrate weak language. The word try will lead to failure. The client must discard the word in order to be able to think positively.

Mind reading
The following are tricks that you may use to dismiss the idea of psychics, albeit you will do this rarely, if ever.

The reader of this should now do the following quickly and spontaneously:
1. Think of an odd number between one and nine.
2. Think of a root vegetable.
3. Imagine you are in a meadow and you look across a stream to the edge of a deep forest. You can see an animal standing there. What is it?
4. Which way is it looking?

I will give the answers and explanations later.

Emotional decision making.
A quick way to help people to make a decision is to toss a coin. You can ask a client what the choices are and then say that you will toss a

coin. If it is a head then choice number one will be the answer, if a tail, then the second option will be chosen. Then toss the coin and tell the client what is on the coin. Then ask, and this is the punch line, whether they were happy or not with the result. If they were happy then that was the right decision, but, if they were saddened then it was the wrong one. This will add an emotional component to their decision making.

They must never follow what the coin suggests as if it were a mystic force, but they follow their reaction to its answer. <u>Then</u> they can make the correct choice.

Aftershocks and panic

Sometimes after the client has gone away from treatment for panic attacks they will feel similar symptoms in some situations. These, I refer to as aftershocks. I will explain that a few wobbly feelings never mean that the problem is coming back but rather that they are like a smaller version of the original problem as it disappears. As, in an earthquake the original shake might be at 8 on the Richter scale, followed by a 5 and then perhaps a 3. This is the original problem settling down. An analogy with a bouncing ball coming to rest serves this purpose as well.

Mind reading answers:

All of the answers are based on the most common spontaneous replies. This is playing a game with odds that are loaded.

1. Most people say seven. After that the number three is second favourite, and then number five.

2. The most popular is carrot followed by potato.

3. It should be a deer. To do this a scene should be set that puts this fairly common animal into the mind. The idea of a meadow and stream will suggest that. The edge of a deep forest excludes farm animals.

4. It should be looking to the left. When we draw animals we tend to start with the head followed by the body. Right handed people, and most left handed ones will start on the left of the paper hence the animal, hopefully deer, is looking to the left in your mental picture.

PART SEVEN
Summing it all up

Perhaps you will now agree that our job is to deal with those two primeval survival systems; the fight-or-flight response and our ability to store fat.

Some alternative therapies have little to do with real life and Freud's theories are models as useful as Meccano in our current lives. They did their best to segment parts of the mind into different boxes. That is to assume that those boxes existed in the first place. If you are afraid to criticise the theories, or hypotheses from a bygone era, and some treatments that are emerging now then you must think again. Rather than accepting something, please examine it, appraise it and if it works then adopt it.

However, we need to offer simplicity in therapy, the problems of our clients are complicated enough to add interest and mystery for the therapist. When therapies become too difficult to even understand the meaning of their names, let-alone the methods of operation, then it is time to really become focussed on what is going to work for the person asking for help. Your clients' aim is to lose a problem. Our aim should be to be of assistance to them without offering to knit fog. We are only here because our clients need help. Please keep it simple. Please keep it effective. Please keep it honest.

Thank you for reading Strictly for Therapists.

John Smale

RECOMMENDED READING

Rather than giving a list of books that might be of use, I would refer you to my website. This is because books can go out of print and new books can be added.

You can find books that I feel are of interest at:

www.emp3books.com/reading.htm

Lightning Source UK Ltd.
Milton Keynes UK
UKOW032239130412

190694UK00001B/53/P